Routledge Revivals

Community Care

When this book was originally published in 1990, the policy of 'community care' occupied a central place in the development of health and social services in Britain. The elderly or mentally ill were being moved out from long-stay hospitals into the community. However, many problems arose from the planning-co-ordination and implementation of this policy and then, as now, community care is at a crisis point. In this book, workers from different areas of community care – the Health Service, voluntary bodies, politics, universities highlight the issues surrounding the run-down of long-stay institutions and make positive suggestions about how individual and agencies can provide effective community care. The contributors examine the political and historical context of community care and discuss whether the move towards care in the community actually improves the quality of life for patients. They look at planning services, and discuss examples of good practice in community care, encouraging practitioners to be more involved in the evaluation of community services. The book will be of interest to a wide range of professionals and voluntary workers in all fields of community care.

Community Care

People Leaving Long-Stay Hospitals

Edited by Sheila Sharkey and Sara Barna

Routledge
Taylor & Francis Group

First published in 1990 by Routledge.

This edition first published in 2026 by Routledge
4 Park Square, Milton Park, Abingdon, Oxon, OX14 4RN

and by Routledge
605 Third Avenue, New York, NY 10158

Routledge is an imprint of the Taylor & Francis Group, an informa business

ISBN: 978-1-041-23663-4 (hbk)
ISBN: 978-1-003-73862-6 (ebk)
ISBN: 978-1-041-23852-2 (pbk)

Book DOI 10.4324/9781003738626

COMMUNITY CARE

People leaving long-stay hospitals

EDITED BY SHEILA SHARKEY
AND SARA BARNA

ROUTLEDGE

First published in 1990 by Routledge
11 New Fetter Lane, London EC4P 4EE

Typeset by LaserScript Limited, Mitcham, Surrey
Printed in Great Britain

British Library Cataloguing in Publication Data

Community care: people leaving long-stay hospitals
1. Great Britain. Community care
I. Sharkey, Sheila II. Barna, Sara
362.1'0425

ISBN 0-415-00609-0

CONTENTS

FIGURES

TABLES

ABBREVIATIONS

APH	Aged persons' home
ATC	Adult Training Centre
CAPE	Clifton Assessment Procedure for the Elderly
CPN	Community Psychiatric Nurse
CPRS	Cambridge Psychiatric Rehabilitation Service
DHSS	Department of Health and Social Security
HA	Health Authority
IDC	Independent Development Council for People with Mental Handicap
NHS	National Health Service
SSD	Social Services Department

ACKNOWLEDGEMENTS

This book is based on a national multidisciplinary conference which was held in Northumberland in June 1987, to which we gave the title 'What do you do after you say goodbye?'. The conference was organized by the Northumberland Health Authority District Psychology Service in conjunction with the Training Section, and we are indebted to many colleagues who made the event possible. First of all we would like to thank Andy Maxwell from the Training Section, who was involved in much of the administrative work of organizing the conference. Our thanks go also to colleagues within the District Psychology Service: Roger Paxton, Paul Smith, and Derek Milne, who acted as chairmen during the conference, and others, in particular Mike Beattie, Lesley Chaplin, Alison Clark, Míchάel Gallagher, Irene Pitt, Nick Radcliffe, and Teresa Wall, who provided invaluable practical help in a variety of ways and also moral support which was much appreciated. The conference participants, many of whom had somewhat arduous journeys, contributed to lively discussions through the three days which have helped to shape this collection of papers. Last but not least, our heartfelt thanks go to Kathleen Kilgour, Barbara Kirkup, and other secretarial staff, who were involved in an enormous amount of work in relation to the original conference, work which has continued with the preparation of this book.

CONTRIBUTORS

Steve Baldwin Principal Clinical Psychologist, General Hospital St. Helier, Jersey, Channel Islands

Sara Barna Principal Clinical Psychologist, Bath Health Authority, formerly Principal Clinical Psychologist, Northumberland Health Authority

Stephen Beyer Mental Handicap in Wales – Applied Research Unit

Roger Blunden Director, King's Fund Centre, London, formerly Director, Mental Handicap in Wales – Applied Research Unit

Frances Brown Co-ordinator, Training Team for Mental Handicap Services, North Western Regional Health Authority

Gerry Evans Mental Handicap in Wales – Applied Research Unit

David Felce Director, British Institute of Mental Handicap

Annette Hames Senior Clinical Psychologist, Community Mental Handicap Team, Newcastle Upon Tyne

Chris Heginbotham Formerly National Director, MIND. Fellow in Health Services Management, Kings Fund College

Jan Hill-Tout Principal Clinical Psychologist, Rhondda Vanguard Service to People with Mental Handicaps

Viv Holt Research Officer, Manchester City Council Housing Department

Mike Illingworth Team Leader Adult Services, Stockport Metropolitan Borough Social Services Department

Ian Macdonald Director of the Mental Handicap Services Unit, BIOSS, Brunel University

Nick Maddocks Senior Social Worker, Manchester City Council, Social Services Department

Mark A. J. O'Callaghan District Psychologist, Basildon and Thurrock Health Authority, Basildon General Hospital, Essex; formerly Co-ordinator of Hollymoor Hospital and Middlewood House (Birmingham and Solihull)

Edna Robinson Acting Sub-Unit Manager, Mental Illness Unit, North Manchester Health Authority

Philip Seed Senior Research Fellow, Department of Social Work, University of Aberdeen

Sheila Sharkey Principal Clinical Psychologist, Northumberland Health Authority

Geoff Shepherd Top Grade Psychologist, Fulbourn Hospital, Cambridge

Renée Short Former Chair of Parliamentary Select Committee for Social Services

Derek Thomas Director, National Development Team for People with a Mental Handicap, London

Stuart Todd Mental Handicap in Wales – Applied Research Unit

INTRODUCTION

SHEILA SHARKEY

In June 1987, the Northumberland District Psychology Service organized a national conference entitled 'What do you do after you say goodbye?'. The aim was to explore some of the issues associated with the contraction of long-stay hospitals and the subsequent development of resources in the community. This book contains the papers presented at the conference. The contributors come from a wide range of settings, including the Health Service, voluntary bodies, politics, and universities, and the papers presented therefore reflect a broad spectrum of viewpoints.

A further aim of the conference was to bring together people who work with different client groups, i.e. the recovering mentally ill, people who are elderly, or who have a mental handicap. The processes involved in developing community resources and the problems associated with the contraction of long-stay hospitals across these client groups are often similar and yet workers from these different fields rarely have the opportunity to learn from one another's experiences.

The book is divided into three sections, which follow the organization of the conference. In the first section, the political and historical context of community care is examined along with the associated concern of whether such a move actually improves the quality of life of service consumers. In his chapter Geoff Shepherd focuses particularly on the recovering mentally ill, but highlights the general concern that in the current enthusiasm for community care, there is now a danger of imposing a community solution as the only alternative available, much as the institutional solution was the only one made available in the past. He argues that our enthusiasm to close hospitals overtakes our concern to provide a good-quality service which is geared towards patient need. Particularly in the case of the recovering mentally ill, hospitals have contracted and patients have been discharged to cheap, poorly run, and poorly serviced resources in the community, where they remain isolated, ignored, and forgotten.

This is in stark contrast to the recommendations made by the Parliamentary Select Committee chaired by Renée Short. They recommended that nobody should be discharged from hospital without a practical individual care plan, jointly devised by all concerned, communicated to all those responsible for its implementation, and with a clear mechanism for monitoring its implementation. They also recommended that the resources be made available for this to happen. How many people working in the field, however, can actually claim this to be their experience? All too often quality services are sacrificed to economic expediency. Wards are closed, patients moved, but a better service is not offered.

How does one ensure that a better-quality service is made available? Roger Blunden argues that this is facilitated by a well-planned service, and in this respect suggests that we have much to learn from commercial organizations, where emphasis is laid on operating according to a clear set of values which inform the way in which the organization is run on a day-to-day basis and which emphasizes that consumer views are a key concern. The latter point was also highlighted by Derek Thomas in the second section of the book, which looks at planning services. He outlines an example of planning which is firmly rooted in direct identification with individual people and their needs. He illustrates a process of service planners learning together with service users about new ways of considering the design of services. It is a specific example but one which could provide a general model for others involved in service design. All too often, however, as Mark O'Callaghn emphasizes, little consumer- influenced planning is done, the institution is simply shifted to the community through management rigidly applying guidelines as issued, for example, in DHSS documents such as 'Better services for the mentally ill'(DHSS, 1975). Facilities and practices in the community often perpetuate the worst of the old institutions without any of their redeeming features.

As institutions contract, many staff who have been trained to work in this environment are often simply relocated in the community. As Frances Brown outlines in her chapter, it is assumed that the skills which they possess will transfer to a different context, and what is more, be considered relevant to it. Staff are often expected to cope with changes in location and conditions of service, as well as shifts in philosophy and attitude, without any support or retraining. Brown clearly illustrates that staff-training issues cannot be ignored or seen in isolation but must be an integral part of overall service planning and development.

In planning community services emphasis is placed on joint planning and in multidisciplinary teams working together. On paper this appears to be a sensible, efficient, and effective solution, but in practice there is often conflict and hostility between the workers from different services and different professions which can bar any useful and productive work. In his chapter Ian Macdonald makes the optimistic assumption that people delivering care to client groups are for the most part attempting to provide the best service possible. He argues that all workers essentially share the same basic set of values, but that they differ in their interpretation of which behaviours express positive or negative values. In interpreting one another's behaviour, workers often mistakenly draw conclusions about one another's values. Macdonald argues that for any joint work to be successful, we must accord the same respect to our colleagues that we accord to our clients. He suggests that any joint work should be led by someone who is able to understand how the different value systems are expressed and enable workers to examine this expression in a secure and accepting environment.

The third and final section of the book it concerned with examples of good practice in relation to community care. It is often easy to overlook such practices in the gloom and despondency which many workers in the field experience. Geoff Shepherd outlines how integrated community and hospital services can be organized and planned for the recovering mentally ill while taking account of some clients' needs for long-term care.

In her chapter on challenging behaviours, Jan Hill-Tout outlines the pioneering approach of the Rhondda Vanguard Service, which, having found that traditional behavioural techniques were limited in their usefulness, had to develop new, person-centred ways of enabling clients with challenging behaviours to become integrated into the community. This example clearly illustrates that effective community care is often costly, requiring a large investment of professional time and expertise.

Because many community-care solutions are expensive, it is imperative in the current climate to demonstrate that clients actually benefit from the solutions. Evaluation of complex and varied solutions is difficult, however. Philip Seed outlines a method of evaluation – social network analysis – which provides a way of evaluating specific services (for example, day centres, domiciliary services, and so on) by focusing on which people, places, and activities are important in daily living. Similarly, Steve Baldwin discusses the concept of neighbourhoods and their use in facilitating the evaluation of community solutions.

Most practitioners recognize the need to evaluate their work in the community, but many feel daunted by the task. Annette Hames outlines how service providers can build evaluation into their everyday practice, and David Felce demonstrates how evaluation can be rigorous and yet unintrusive in a community setting.

Overall this book is an attempt to highlight some of the issues surrounding the run-down of long-stay institutions. As such it contains a message of hope and a warning – as Chris Heginbotham says, community care is at a crisis point, in danger of getting a bad name – not because it has failed, but rather because it has still hardly started. Our hope is that this book will point out some of the pitfalls of the process and offer some suggestions as to how individuals and agencies can actually get started.

REFERENCE

DHSS (1975) *Better Services for the Mentally Ill*, London: HMSO

Part One

THE CONTEXT OF CARE IN THE COMMUNITY

Chapter One

THE POLITICAL CONTEXT OF CARE IN THE COMMUNITY

A review of the work of the parliamentary select committee for social services

RENÉE SHORT

The Select Committee decided in the 1984 Session of Parliament to look at the problems of caring for adult mentally ill and mentally handicapped people. Mental illness affects people of every level of intelligence. Their illness can very often improve with treatment or clear up completely. Mental handicap, on the other hand, is nearly always present from birth or early childhood. It is irreversible although its effects can be ameliorated by training, by environmental influences, and by the right contacts. Some mentally handicapped people suffer from mental illness and some mentally ill people are in effect handicapped when their disorders are severe. All of them need some privacy, and they may need protection from others and from themselves. Thus, although the two categories are often considered separately, the conclusions for both groups are often very similar. In our enquiry, which dealt only with adults, we decided to use the phrase 'mentally disabled' to cover both mentally handicapped and mentally ill people.

Community care is often used in misleading ways. It does not mean:

(1) saving money on the cost of hospital care by getting people out of hospital,
(2) nor care by families or volunteers rather than statutory care,
(3) nor the transfer of responsibility from the NHS to local authorities.

Some general principles can help us to define it:

(1) the preference for home life over institutional care;
(2) the need for integration in a normal background, avoiding as far as possible segregation and restriction;

(3) small is often better than large;
(4) local services are better than remote ones.

The aim should therefore be to enable individuals to lead as normal a life as possible, with the minimum disruption within their community, while taking into account their particular disabilities. This then means that wherever possible, people with mental disability should live in ordinary housing, should – if possible – have some occupation and should be able to use ordinary recreational facilities. This means that care must be provided in many different locations which may include hospitals. The local health and social authorities have the responsibility of assessing patients' needs, of providing necessary treatment and care, and, where necessary, allocating suitable environments. If disruption is to be minimized, it is also necessary to help families, to support them, and to deal with special problems as they occur. Perhaps even more important, it is necessary to educate members of the general community about the problems affecting the mentally disabled and their families, so that they can help as well.

In 1984 our committee went to the United States. We found more varied provision than in the UK and a much greater participation of private psychiatric practice than in the UK. We visited one large State mental hospital with about 20,000 patients and I think it is true to say that this offered a lower standard of care than a large hospital in the UK.

However, we learned one very important lesson from the US – namely, that however imperfect the facilities for patients in hospital may be, you cannot close these down until better facilities are very firmly established. There is no merit in moving patients from a large mental hospital to cheaper, less well staffed institutions, whether you call them nursing homes or community homes. Such moves may help us to close hospitals but it does not really help patients.

In Nebraska we saw an excellent example of co-operation between employers and trade unions in order to provide work for former patients. We visited a large engineering works where part of the shop-floor had been set aside for former patients, both men and women. They were trained in the use of machines and were turning out small parts. They had been trained on the job and they received the rate for the job and we were told there had been no problems with the rest of the work-force or their trade unions.

Moreover, all these former patients were living out in the community, with their families, and all of them said they had been accepted by their neighbours. We also met a group of four former patients, young women living with their caring staff in an attractive modern house, in a typical middle-class American suburb. The house was well furnished and some of the young women went to a training centre or to other neighbourhood activities. They, too, had had no problems with their neighbours.

In Italy the number of in-patients halved between 1961 and 1978 and then, after an energetic campaign by Psichiatrica Democratica, admissions and readmissions to mental hospitals were forbidden and the funding of hospitals ceased, even though there were thousands of long-stay patients still in them. There is no specialized day care and the new community health centres are not very good, so that public opinion is against these so-called reforms. There are important lessons for us to learn from both the US and Italian examples.

I must disabuse anyone who thinks that community care can be cost neutral. If we think of the growing numbers of mentally disabled people living in the community with older parents, it is clear that some additional provision will have to be made for them. What are we to do for the thousands of mentally ill or handicapped people still living in the large, inadequate Victorian hospitals? Are we to continue to devote scarce resources to shoring them up at increasing capital and revenue cost or should we demolish them and replace them by suitable housing and caring staff at even greater expense? If we decide to keep the hospitals, then quite clearly staffing ratios and the proportion of trained staff available would certainly have to be improved.

At the present time we are providing a mental disability service which is under-financed and under-staffed both in its health and social aspects. Community care on the cheap is worse in many respects than what we already provide in the large hospitals and the Minister of State at that time admitted to us that 'if you have a hospital facility which in the past has been greatly under-funded, if you transfer the function to community care, the costs will go up.'

The Committee told the Government that genuine community care can only be achieved with some real increase in expenditure over a period of years for mentally disabled patients.

In the long term we would expect to see a reduction in expenditure by health authorities and an increase in local authority expenditure in terms of education, housing, and transport, and this is the message that runs right through our report. There would be a greater burden placed on voluntary organizations, relatives, and families and certainly on the social security budget, for as patients leave hospital, their individual social security entitlements are most probably going to be their major source of finance, as they are for those at present in the community.

The Committee visited several regions during our enquiry and from what we saw of many local authorities, it was clear that they seemed to regard social security as a bottomless pit. If the Government is prepared to provide the resources – which is what we told them to do – well and good, but if the Government wishes to put the lid on social security payments, then mentally disabled people may become very vulnerable.

The minister told us that there had certainly been an escalation of costs in this area and there has been considerable growth of private homes catering for former patients which are run at a profit. He said, 'we have to take a view of the totality of spending and my colleagues have taken the view there should be ministerial control on this.'

The reduction in the number of in-patients beds that has taken place so far has certainly made it more difficult for patients requiring psychiatric in-patient treatment. Parents of schizophrenic patients especially find it more and more difficult to get a bed. The police also complain of difficulties in getting admission for mentally disordered people who come into custody. Consultant psychiatrists told us that when staff are absent through sickness they very often have to refuse admission, and general practitioners also told us of similar difficulties. There is no doubt that very great strain is put on the families of mentally ill people. The Committee recommended that catchment areas of mental illness hospitals should be more flexible and that admission policies should be based on an individual's need for treatment or care. We are horrified that patients are still being discharged unable to cope with day-to-day living and as the National Schizophrenia Fellowship told us, many 'are on park benches, in prisons, doss houses, or seedy and rapacious lodgings.' Suicides are not unusual.

Of course, therefore, the Committee recommended that nobody should be discharged from hospital without a practical individual care plan jointly devised by all concerned, communicated to all those responsible for its implementation, and with a mechanism for monitoring its implementation or its modification, in the light of changing conditions, and that resources for this be made available.

As the mental-handicap hospitals are run down, the mentally handicapped will need good social provision and, of course, some medical care. In Omaha we visited the University Psychiatric Institute which provides back-up for the community services and these were provided for former patients living in ordinary housing. We saw something similar at St Abba's but there are few such models available. The Committee urged the Department and the professions to co-operate in the production of practical options for medical services in the context of locally based community care.

We visited the Rudolf Steiner Settlement on the shores of Belfast Lough for about sixty mentally handicapped children and thirty adults. There are many craft activities and excellent workshops, a lovely weaving shop and a splendid, well-run farm, including cattle breeding. Many of the carers come from abroad, many of them are Quakers, many are followers of Rudolf Steiner. They have close contacts with the surrounding community and there is a very wide range of choice for mentally handicapped people there.

I would like to conclude by saying some cautionary words about the growth of private provision for former mentally disabled patients. Widespread concern was expressed to us about this, both that provided in ordinary houses and in larger residential institutions. According to figures supplied by the DHSS, the numbers do not appear to be large at the moment, roughly about 2000 places in 131 premises, about double what it was ten years ago. The DHSS told us that about one-third of mentally disabled people financially supported by local authorities are in private or voluntary homes. In Norfolk and Lancashire, Worcester and Hereford, and in North East London great anxiety about private residential care was expressed to us.

We recommended that local authorities should be able to designate and inspect private homes. We also recommended the example set in Norfolk, where registration has been made into an educative process and where aspiring proprietors are obliged to attend and pay for training courses. Proper inspection and registration can maintain standards. The ultimate sanction for unsatisfactory proprietors is de-registration, but then of course, alternative accommodation has to be found for the inmates, often at very short notice.

The concerns that were raised with us are very real and recent legislation has not really solved the problem. We told the Secretary of State to review this again, but in any case, there should be a review of the principles and procedures governing the vetting of applicants to run private homes.

Voluntary organisations, like MENCAP, MIND, the Spastics Society, the Campaign for Mentally Handicapped people, NSF, the Richmond Fellowship, the National Autistic Society, the Mental Health Foundation, the National Council for Voluntary Organizations, the Standing Conference for Voluntary Organizations in Wales, the Salvation Army, CHAR, and many other voluntary organizations do sterling work in this field and General Practitioners, of course have a very important role to play. They relieve the Government to a very considerable extent by providing services that are very often better and cheaper than the Government can provide themselves.

We are very keen to see greater practical recognition of the value of the voluntary sector. They are very often more willing to include the participation of parents and relatives in planning and managing their services. The Government is always happy to pay lip-service to the work of the voluntary bodies but they are not always willing to provide adequate grants to encourage innovation or particularly effective projects. The other problem is that they are short-term. The Committee told the Department to look at this again and to be more flexible in funding.

Chapter Two

COMMUNITY CARE

A historical overview

GEOFF SHEPHERD

INTRODUCTION

It was A. J. P. Taylor, writing of Napoleon, who said that he was a student of history, and like most of those who study history, he learned from the mistakes of the past how to make new ones. I sometimes think that there must be a lot of very fine historians amongst our current crop of planners and managers since, with or without the benefit of much historical knowledge, they seem pretty determined to repeat most of the mistakes that have already been made in the history of community care and to add a few more of their own. It is my aim in this chapter to try and identify some of these lessons of history in the hope that an awareness of their existence will reduce the likelihood that they will be committed again in the future. I have to say that I am not particularly hopeful about achieving my aim.

THE LESSONS OF HISTORY

1. Those with long-term social and psychiatric problems – like the poor – are always with us and they present very special problems for a service built around notions like 'patients', 'treatments', 'cure', and so on.

The problems of the long-term mentally ill are not a new invention. Historical records of seventeenth-century physicians show a similar range of psychological disorders to those that we are familiar with today (MacDonald 1983). There were anxiety states, obsessional disorders, depression – actually quite a common and rather fashionable malady – in addition to those suffering from the more severe forms of lunacy characterized by bursts of frantic energy, restless wandering, fits of wildly inappropriate laughter and 'verbal pandemonium' (talking in an incoherent or tormented fashion). It is also apparent that these more severe conditions were considerably rarer than the more common disturbances of mood and emotion, just as they are today.

Of course, the reactions of physicians like Richard Napier, who is the subject of Michael MacDonald's book, were rather different from their modern counterparts. Napier was an eclectic and he mixed medical, religious, even magical remedies according to what he thought would suit his patients. He sought to cure the body and, at the same time, to soothe the spirit. It was not until 200 years later that these approaches were replaced by the narrow, somatic views of the Victorian 'mad-doctors'. Napier also never used institutional care: he worked entirely 'in the community' because there was no other option.

By the nineteenth century the situation had changed: the mental hospitals had been built in the hope that they would provide a *cure* for mental illness and that once successfully treated the patients would not return. There was therefore considerable dismay when it began to be realized that there was a steady build-up of 'chronic' and 'incurable' cases in the new asylums. To use Alexander Leighton's vivid phrase, 'the cult of curability was replaced by the incubus of incurability' (Leighton 1982). Various schemes were then put forward as to how to deal with these problems – for example, admit only treatable cases to the institutions and provide custodial care, at a much lower cost, in the community for the more chronic cases (Caton 1984: 11). The term 'surplus insane' was also coined to describe these difficult and recalcitrant cases.

'Surplus' to what?, you might well ask. 'Surplus', I would suggest, to a system of care which relied for its rationale on notions of 'sickness', 'treatment', and 'cure'. Being a 'patient' should be a temporary condition. You get ill, you receive treatment (take your medicine) and you get better. While you are 'ill' you are excused the normal duties and responsibilities of life; when you get better you have to take them up again. Thus, the idea of a *chronic* patient is a contradiction in terms. You cannot be a proper patient and be untreatable at the same time; it just does not make sense. It also becomes difficult to justify the expenditure of scarce, therapeutic resources on people who are not going to get better. This is undoubtedly a part of the reason why chronic patients do not receive their fair share of resources – nor are likely to – in a health system in which success is measured by 'cure' rates or numbers discharged. One cannot help wondering what their fate might have been had they fallen into some other system of care – for example, one with a religious or political ideology.

Thus, chronic patients present a problem. They are an embarrassment to a scientific and technological culture which is used to being able to sort out its problems. It is not surprising then that they should have attracted a wide range of different solutions and that each new solution should have been greeted with such desperate enthusiasm.

2. From time to time people have thought they had found an answer to these complex social and psychiatric problems; at one time this was to build institutions; now it is to close them.

The institutions were not built as a place for dumping poor and inadequate individuals who were not coping in society and who embarrassed genteel sensibilities (although they may have come to fulfil this function later in their history). They were built because people believed they would provide an effective way of *curing* mental illness. Heavily influenced by the example of the York Retreat, the new asylums were built as models of the very latest knowledge in the treatment of mental disorder, and pioneer reformers like Dorothea Dix travelled the world persuading people that they *must* build institutions. She believed that if treatment could be given early enough then cure was 'inevitable' and that it was only the neglected cases that became incurable. Thus, in 1845, she dared the legislature of Nova Scotia 'to refuse what you *know* will heal the sick' (cited in Leighton 1982: 25). Thus, why did the asylums 'fail'?

There were many reasons (see Shepherd 1984: Chapter 2). These included increased size and overcrowding, inadequate resources, decreased staffing levels, changes in legislation, changing theoretical attitudes towards the role of social factors in aetiology and care, and, possibly most importantly of all, an attempt to apply the model to inappropriate populations. Thus, the York Retreat, where the techniques of moral treatment were developed, was a small, private institution where most of the residents were from middle or upper class backgrounds. By contrast, the public institutions were having to deal with large numbers of poor and ill-educated people, drawn to the cities by the Industrial Revolution, and also the increasing numbers of elderly who were living longer as a result of the general improvement in health standards. 'Moral treatment' may not therefore have failed; it may simply have been evaluated with insufficient regard to the 'specificity' of its effects. Now, there is a lesson for our modern planners and researchers.

In any event, after barely fifty years people had lost faith – and by and large also lost interest – in institutional solutions. By the turn of the century they were looking again to 'community care' to provide the answer and this time they were armed with the new psychological treatments like psychoanalysis and new ideas like the 'Mental Hygiene' movement which involved for the first time a coalition of 'consumers' and professionals. The emphasis thus shifted towards prevention and early intervention in the community, on stopping people going into hospital, rather than caring for them once they got in there. These ideas were already well established by the inter-war period (see Jones 1972: Chapter 9), but they did not become national policy until the 1959 Mental Health Act and the subsequent 1962 Hospital Plan (DHSS 1962). Since then successive governments have tried to shift the location of care away from the mental hospital and towards acute care in district general hospital units and long-term care in the 'community', hopefully being provided by Social Services, private and voluntary agencies, and families.

In some respects it has been a very successful policy. The number of beds in mental hospitals has been halved in twenty-five years (from over 150,000 to less than 70,000). However, although most districts now have a general hospital psychiatric unit, the build-up of community services has been slow and uneven. There is a particular shortage of long-term day support and a worrying recent increase in privately run residential homes funded by social security benefits (House of Commons 1985; Audit Commission 1986). The intended shift towards local authority provision simply has not materialized and there has been more 'trans-institutionalization' than 'de-institutionalization'. Despite the pressure on mental hospitals to close (currently about one-third are due to go by the end of the decade), it has also become increasingly clear that there are substantial numbers of people for whom hospital care – or something very like it – may be a necessity for the foreseeable future. These include both the 'hard core', 'old' long-stay who constitute perhaps a third of the remaining mental hospital population and the small number of 'new' long-stay inpatients who are still accumulating. Thus, talk of 'hospital-hostels' (Wykes 1982), a 'Haven' for the old long-stay to be rebuilt on an existing hospital site (Wing and Furlong 1986), and the use of the mental hospital as a base for a district service if it is 'suitably situated' (DHSS 1985: Annex 1) suggest something of a retreat from the polarized 'anti-hospital' stance of the early sixties.

The impetus behind these changes in the patterns of service delivery has been based on two premisses: first, a belief that care in the community would be more effective than care in hospital, and second, a belief that care in the community would be cheaper. This coalition of therapeutic radicals with fiscal conservatives has proved very powerful, not only in this country but also in many others around the world. However, the debate about 'institutional' versus 'community' care has never been an empirical one; it has always been ideological. People *knew* which was best and they were not going to bother to wait around and collect some evidence to check out their preconceptions. Just like Dorothea Dix, they believed that the superiority of community care was 'inevitable'. It is like a Eurovision song contest with two entrants, where the judges hear the first song and immediately vote for the second! Can we now therefore identify some of the characteristics of a good quality of care that might apply irrespective of its location?

3. Since the beginning, the heart of good quality care has consisted in an attempt to foster a sympathetic interest in, and respect for, the problems of individuals and an emphasis on the importance of the everyday activities of life, rather than complex medical – or psychological – remedies.

A concern and respect for the problems of the individual has been the cornerstone of good-quality care from the days of the York Retreat to the insights of Goffman into 'total institutions' (Goffman 1961) and the empirical work of King et al. (1971), Shepherd and Richardson (1979), and others. Thus, the Italian reformer Chiarugi, writing towards the end of the eighteenth century, stated that, 'It is a supreme moral duty and medical obligation to respect the insane individual as a person' (cited in

Digby 1985: 30). Similarly, Samuel Tuke, the founder of the York Retreat, stated as the central principle of moral treatment that, 'the patient on all occasions should be spoken to and treated as much in the manner of a rational being as the state of his mind will possibly allow' (Hunter and MacAlpine 1965).

Of course, moral treatment did not simply consist of a passive acceptance of the patient and his or her difficulties. The Quaker philosophy believed in regularity, good order, and a 'core belief' that one's life was one's testimony. Everyday activities like conversing with other people, preparing food, looking after your appearance, finding constructive ways to pass the time, and so on, thus became the overriding goals of treatment. They were not peripheral activities, they were the central preoccupation and their value stemmed from their direct tie to 'normal' life and the lives of ordinary people. This 'normalizing' philosophy is very clearly illustrated in the practices of the York Retreat and the early asylum movement (see Jones 1972; Digby 1985). Unfortunately, it was to disappear with the impact of scientific ideas and the shift from a social to a somatic view of mental illness. 'Scientific' (and psychological) theories stressed the importance of understanding and treating peoples' pathology, rather than helping them live their ordinary lives. Those with long-term – and largely untreatable – problems have thereby been locked into a 'sick' role from which there has been little escape. Only recently, perhaps there may be some light at the end of the tunnel.

The same argument applies to the role of work and structured activities in the rehabilitation of those with serious, long-term disorders. Work was seen to be important by the early asylum builders because it provided a way of distracting the mind from 'painful and injurious associations' (Jones 1972: 107). This reflected their strong belief in 'associationist' theories of mind (a belief which, albeit in other forms, I sense that we still hold today). Work was thus considered to be important in its own right, not simply because of its link to financial rewards. Again, this is important to stress in the present climate, where the value of work is liable to be overlooked because of the difficulties of finding paid employment. The pioneers of moral treatment were also committed to providing a range of work from 'the sciences, fine arts, literature or mechanical arts...(to)...drawing, painting, gardening and other means of innocent amusement' (ibid.). I wonder if we have the same commitment to providing such a range of work opportunities today?

4. In the field of mental health provision, there has been a consistent tendency to drift away from those with more difficult problems towards those with less serious disorders.

My next point reminds me of Ralf Dahrendorf's famous dictum that 'history proceeds by changing the subject'. So it has been with the care of the long-term mentally ill. We have seen already how when people began to lose faith in the curative value of the institution, they switched attention to a new set of problems and a new range of treatments outside the hospitals. Similarly, when the new Community Mental Health Centres were created in the Kennedy era in the United States, they were meant to provide an alternative to care in the State hospitals, but they soon gravitated towards providing out-patient services for people who would have been unlikely ever to be admitted to hospital (Mollica 1983). In the UK, the Joint Finance money which was made available in the late seventies to facilitate the run-down of the mental hospitals was used instead to build up services to prevent patients already in the community from having to go into hospital. Thus , in 1983 the DHSS was forced to specifically earmark the 'Care in the Community' money for moving patients out of hospital. Why has there been this consistent drift away from the most disabled and seriously handicapped individuals?

Leighton (1982) argues that there is a specific fear of those with long-term mental illness which distorts society's response to them, leading to denial, repression, and so on. Certainly, chronic patients are an anomaly in treatment-oriented service, and there does seem to be something very deep-rooted in the reaction of successive generations to the problems of those with long-term disorders. Perhaps it is because they are supposed to be 'unrewarding' to work with; perhaps it stems from a failure to identify them clearly enough as a special group with special needs; perhaps it is the fact that the number of professionals who actually have direct experience of working with long-term patients at any one time is rather small and is generally limited to those working in hospital settings.

Whatever the reason, it is clear that a very important task of staff training remains to be done. If most of the expertise and experience lies with staff in institutional settings, it is not surprising that when money gets transferred to the community it tends to be spent on people who the workers 'out there' are most familiar with. These are, by and large, not the people who are likely to spend long periods of time in hospital. If the professionals are only trained to deal with those who have neurotic disorders, then this is who they will wish to treat. If we want them to deal with people who have more chronic problems, then we must train them accordingly. This means teaching them about the principles of rehabilitation, the value of medication, the importance of counselling, and so on. It is therefore a source of constant disappointment to me that psychologists seem extremely interested in developing methods to help people manage chronic physical conditions like diabetes, yet relatively disinterested in the management of chronic psychiatric conditions like schizophrenia.

5. There are fundamental problems in funding a service which is not built around beds.

This brings me to another fundamental lesson: although the mental hospitals have reduced considerably in size, nevertheless they have kept most of the money. Thus, staffing ratios in the institutions have actually *improved* in recent years as unit costs have risen (Audit Commission 1986), and we have the paradoxical situation in which the move towards care in the community has probably benefited the hospitals more than it has the services outside them. The mechanisms for transferring money from Health to Social Services budgets have met with little success mainly because Social Service departments have been reluctant to enter into long-term revenue commitments for fear that they will not be able to meet the 'tapering ' arrangements. The House of Commons Committee (1985) thus regard Joint Finance as 'virtually played out' as a mechanism for transferring funds from NHS to local authorities (para. 108). Whether or not the Audit Commission's recent recommendation to create a single authority responsible for services for the long- term mentally ill proves to be effective, we will have to wait and see.

Ironically, the most successful mechanism for transferring money from the hospital to the community has been the changes in personal social security benefits introduced in 1980 (the so-called '9/5 monies'). As indicated earlier, these have funded the recent boom in private and voluntary residential care with all the problems in monitoring standards that has entailed. The dangers of 'trans-institutionalization', and a community service in which only the residential component is adequately funded, are obvious. Nevertheless, the principle that funding should be tied to the individual, rather than the service, seems to be a sound one.

Of course, the problem of transferring funds from hospital to community is not just confined to the UK. There are similar difficulties throughout Europe and in the USA (Mangen 1985; Jansen 1987). We therefore need a new system for calculating funding which is not based on beds. My own preference would be for cars per 100,000 of the population since this would reflect the transition towards a much more mobile, community-based service. We could have 'x' acute cars, 'y' chronic cars, 'z' psychogeriatric cars, and so on.

6. The mental hospitals were invented because the public wanted a system which was open and accountable and in which, if there were abuses occurring, then people would know about them.

Finally, we must consider the monitoring and evaluation of services. The mental hospitals were built partly because people were concerned about the abuses that were occurring in the private madhouses. Now that we are moving once again towards a multi-agency, multi-site service, the questions of inspection and monitoring of standards must be addressed. The issue is not whether abuses will occur, for surely they will. Such is the darker side of human nature and that certainly does not change. The issue is how we can ensure that, as far as possible, we will become aware of these abuses. Much has been said and written about how to achieve a good 'quality of care' and it seems to me now high time to get on with implementing some of these recommendations. This means setting up monitoring groups, working with local MIND organizations, the Community Health Councils, inviting in independent advocates, and so on. Everybody knows that we will not improve the quality of care simply by changing its location. If we are not to see a return to abuses of a dispersed and highly variable service of 200 years ago, we must set up adequate systems of inspection and monitoring now.

CONCLUSIONS

I have tried to identify some of the historical lessons. I would like to think that we will learn from our mistakes, but I remain sceptical. Of course, my list is not an exhaustive one, but one fact stands out.

The mental hospital was 'invented' in an attempt to meet the needs of some very disadvantaged and disabled people and simply abolishing the hospitals will not eliminate those needs. As Leona Bachrach (1978) has reminded us, institutions fulfil a range of social functions (asylum, treatment, occupation, social support, the provision of a secure environment, and a source of employment for a variety of professionals), in addition to their very limited role of providing long-term accommodation. If we have ambitions to do away with the mental hospital, we therefore have to think how we are going to meet all of these needs in different ways in the community. In doing so we must not confuse reducing people's *handicaps*, i.e. their social disadvantages, with managing their *disabilities*, i.e. helping them live with relatively fixed difficulties in social role performance.

The key ingredient in all this will, of course, be people. From the York Retreat to the present day, the history of caring for the long-term mentally ill has been studded with the names of outstanding individuals – Tuke, Connolly, Clark, Bennett, Wing, et al. There have also been many people whose names never find their way into the history books, but whose dedication and compassion have made these services work. People are always more important than money (though this is not to say that money is not important too!), but leadership, vision, and commitment remain the essential ingredients of change.

REFERENCES

Audit Commission (1986) *Making a Reality of Community Care*, London: HMSO.

Bachrach, L. L. (1978) 'A conceptual approach to deinstitutionalisation', *Hospital and Community Psychiatry* 29: 573–8.

Caton, C. (1984) *Management of Chronic Schizophrenia*, New York: Oxford University Press.

Department of Health and Social Security (1962) *Hospital Plan for England and Wales*, Cmnd. 1604, London: HMSO.

Department of Health and Social Security (1985) 'Mental illness: policies for prevention, treatment, rehabilitation and care, Annex 1' to *Government Response to the Second Report from the Social Services Committee 1984–85*, Cmnd. 9624, London: HMSO.

Digby, A. (1985) *Madness, Morality and Medicine: A Study of the York Retreat 1796–1910*, Cambridge: Cambridge University Press.

Goffman, E. (1961) *Asylums*, Doubleday, New York: Anchor Books.

House of Commons (1985) *Second Report from the Social Services Committee on Community Care*, London: HMSO.

Hunter, R. and MacAlpine, I. (1965) 'Samual Tuke's first publication in the treatment of patients at the retreat', *British Journal of Psychiatry* 111: 771–8.

Jansen, M. A. (1987) *An International Perspective on Community Services and Rehabilitation for Persons with Chronic Mental Illness*, Monograph Number 36, New York: World Rehabilitation Fund.

Jones, K. (1972) *A History of the Mental Health Services*, London: Routledge & Kegan Paul.

King, R., Raynes, N. and Tizard, J. (1971) *Patterns of Residential Care*, London: Routledge & Kegan Paul.

Leighton, A. (1982) *Caring for Mentally Ill People*, Cambridge: Cambridge University Press.

MacDonald, M. (1983) *Mystical Bedlam: Madness, Anxiety and Healing in Seventeenth Century England*, Cambridge: Cambridge University Press.

Mangen, S. (1985) *Mental Health Care in the European Community*, London: Croom Helm.

Mollica, R. F. (1983) 'From asylum to community: the threatened disintegration of public psychiatry', *New England Journal of Medicine* 308: 367–73.

Shepherd, G. (1984) *Institutional Care and Rehabilitation*, London: Longmans.

——and Richardson, A. (1979) 'Organisation and interaction in psychiatric day centres', *Psychological Medicine* 9: 573–9.

Wing, J. K. and Furlong, R. (1986) 'A haven for the severely disabled within the context of a comprehensive psychiatric community service', *British Journal of Psychiatry* 149: 449–57.

Wykes, T. (1982) 'A hostel-ward for 'new' long-stay patients', in J. K. Wing (ed.) *Long-term community Care: Experience in a London Borough*, Psychological Medicine Monograph Supplement Number 2, Cambridge: Cambridge University Press.

Chapter Three

SAFEGUARDING QUALITY

ROGER BLUNDEN

The current movement towards the development of community services for people with learning disabilities has stemmed from a concern to extend the quality of life of individual service users. Service plans now often include an explicit commitment to treat users on an individual basis and to work towards improving their life-styles. This is also reflected in the development of methods of 'individual planning' (see, for example, Blunden 1980), which are designed to help professionals and others co-ordinate their activities around the lives of individual users. It is clear that the development of new services is itself a learning experience. There are no ready answers to key questions about how services should be designed and implemented. We have seen a diversity of schemes set up in various parts of Britain, each involving a creative local response to the problems of providing effective services. As the Audit Commission (1986) made clear, examples of good practice are often the result of action by strong and committed local 'champions' of change.

It is important, therefore, that not only do we create the conditions which will enable such local initiatives to flourish, but that we also provide safeguards to ensure that quality, once achieved, is maintained. This highlights a need to ensure that service development becomes a *dynamic* process. There needs to be built in to the 'system' a capacity for rectifying weaknesses and making further improvements. This chapter explores ways in which those providing services can constantly question what they are doing, learn from their experience, and incorporate these lessons into practice.

Although most people would agree that services for people with learning disabilities should be of a high quality, it is not always particularly clear what we mean by 'a high-quality service'. Different people may well have different notions of quality. A useful starting-point is therefore to clarify just what a quality service might look like in practice. In this discussion we are concerned with a wide range of community-based services, such as those which support people in their own homes, provide access to education, work or leisure, or which support people with learning disabilities in residential accommodation in the community. Whilst all these forms of service provision have different aims, there are some characteristics which quality services might be expected to have in common.

ACCESSIBILITY

One important set of characteristics come under the heading of 'accessibility'. Does a particular form of service exist locally? How easy is it for users to find out about it? Is it easy to contact? Is it located within easy reach? Is there sufficient service to meet users' demand for it? Are the staff welcoming, friendly, and helpful?

These aspects of service quality are all vitally important. Many problems with existing services stem from deficiencies in accessibility: for example, there are gaps in service provision. Many parts of the UK do not have adequate respite services, or the availability of community residential services is limited, or there is a very limited range of further education available to people with learning disabilities. Often specialist services such as speech therapy or physiotherapy are in short supply. Where a service does exist, it may be remote, difficult to contact, or not be particularly welcoming to users. From recent discussions with families with a disabled member it is clear that many experience just these sorts of difficulties when dealing with some DHSS offices. They have great difficulty in finding out their eligibility for benefits, and in some cases have to go to extraordinary lengths to obtain their entitlement. These examples contrast with the notion of an accessible service, readily available and offering a welcoming face to its users.

EFFECTIVENESS

Whilst all these features are important characteristics of a service's quality, they say nothing about the effectiveness of the service in meeting its users' needs. Even where a service exists locally and is readily accessible, this is no guarantee that it is effectively resolving the problems which its users present. There is perhaps an analogy with other services, such as a solicitor's offices. It may be there, offer ready appointments, and have a friendly receptionist, but this says nothing about its ability to offer effective legal advice.

In this discussion of service quality, we are particularly concerned with effectiveness. In developing community services we have understandably placed a great deal of emphasis on ensuring that services are available and accessible to local users. However, it is equally important that attention is devoted to the effectiveness of these services.

So what is 'effectiveness' in the context of services for people with learning disabilities? Because services aim to help people with almost every aspect of life, it is often quite difficult to give a specific answer to this question. However, one useful view of service aims has been set out by John O'Brien (1987). O'Brien suggests that there are five important ways in which services for people with learning disabilities should affect their users' lives. These are:

(1) *Community presence.* Services should enable their users to live and spend time within their local community, not segregated from other people. This applies to all aspects of life – home, work, education, leisure. One measure of a service's effectiveness would be the extent to which its users spend their time in settings where they have the opportunity to mix with other non-handicapped people.

(2) *Relationships.* As well as providing the opportunities for people with learning disabilities to mix with other people, services will be effective to the extent that their users are helped to form relationships with other people in society.

(3) *Choice.* An effective service will also extend the range of choices available to those who use it. In the past, services have often restricted the choices available to their users, both in terms of everyday decisions like what to eat or what to wear, and over more major life events such as where and with whom to live.

(4) *Competence.* Because people have learning disabilities, an effective service will support its users in learning and making use of new skills, relevant to their living situation. Thus, service users should experience a growing ability to perform useful and meaningful activities, with whatever assistance is required.

(5) *Respect.* It has often been the case that people with learning disabilities have been treated as second-class citizens and denied the respect that is afforded to most members of society. Effective services will seek to reverse this process and ensure that their users are promoted as valued people in their own right.

These five aspects of life provide a useful starting-point for a discussion of service effectiveness. They help pinpoint ways in which we might expect to see quality services influencing the lives of those who use them. They are in line with the original principles of the *An Ordinary Life* initiative and give a practical basis for examining service effectiveness.

LESSONS FROM COMMERCIAL ORGANIZATIONS

Of course the issue of quality is not unique to services for people with learning disabilities. Other organizations face the same problems of attempting to keep abreast of change, adapting to a changing environment and keeping their 'customers' satisfied. In essence a service for people with learning disabilities faces many of the same challenges as a commercial company. The organization has to justify its existence. In commercial terms this usually means making a profit. In the case of a service, this profit motive may be replaced by a concern to benefit the users of the service, or at least to avoid causing them harm. In the field of learning disabilities the concern in the past has often been to avoid the scandals which have arisen due to some of the worst examples of neglect. However, the acceptance by some of the more positive philosophy of 'an ordinary life' has lead to more critical questioning of the aims and achievements of service systems.

Beyond simply justifying their existence, many people seek to maximize the effectiveness of the organization for which they work. This implies a constant questioning of whether the best is being achieved with the resources available. As new methods of working are developed, there is a concern to incorporate these into the way in which the service is delivered.

In recent years a great deal has been written about the pursuit of quality in the context of commercial organizations. Indeed, at the present time, there is something of a cult in books offering advice on the pursuit of excellence. These draw on the experience gained in a range of commercial companies and highlight key features of successful organizations. One of these books, *In Search of Excellence* (Peters and Waterman 1982), draws attention to a number of characteristics of successful commercial organizations. Although there may not be a direct comparison between US commercial companies and services for people with learning disabilities in Britain, *In Search of Excellence* does describe an organizational culture in which quality is promoted in a number of ways. It is perhaps useful to picture the sort of service organization which would mirror the vision of a successful, quality conscious, corporation.

The quality conscious service would have an explicit set of values, informing the way in which the organization ran on a day-by-day basis. These values would emphasize the importance of the service consumer (the 'customer'). There would be an obsession with quality, in terms of meeting consumers' needs throughout the organization – from the most senior managers to front-line workers. Managers at all levels would make a point of maintaining contact with service consumers, treating their views and problems as items of key concern. The focus of the organization would be on results, not process. The organizational structure would be fluid in nature, with small groups and task-forces being formed around the solution of particular problems. The formal structure of the organization would not be allowed to get in the way of achieving results. Staff would be actively encouraged to innovate and to champion new ideas. There would be recognition that not all new ideas would succeed – failure would be tolerated and lessons learned from the experience. Peters and Waterman create the image of a highly motivated work- force, being given ample scope and encouragement to pursue the clearly defined aims of the organization. They use the term 'simultaneous tight-loose properties' to describe the way in which people within the organization are given maximum individual autonomy within the context of firm central direction.

Many services present a very different picture form this image of an accessible action-oriented and quality-conscious organization. Is this an unrealistic vision, or are there ways in which this notion of quality can be built into the ways in which services for people with learning disabilities are organized and delivered?

PURSUING QUALITY WITHIN SERVICE ORGANIZATIONS

One set of ideas for helping to ensure that quality is 'built in' to the service system has recently been promoted by the Independent Development Council for People with Mental Handicap in their booklet *Pursuing Quality* (IDC 1986). This sets out to provide practical guidance to people concerned with service quality. The IDC start by assuming that a number of conditions will need to be met if a service is effectively to review its quality and take steps to improve it. The first is that key 'stakeholders' should be involved in defining and reviewing service quality. A stakeholder is anyone with a major interest in the service in question. Stakeholders are likely to include service users, family members, front-line staff, other professionals and managers; and may also involve representatives of the wider community such as local residents or politicians. It is argued that all these people have a key interest in the quality of the service and will be directly affected by attempts to produce change. Their active participation will help ensure that their interests are respected and will thus help ensure that any decisions made are more likely to be put into practice.

The second feature of an effective approach to service quality is that the service should be based upon a clear statement of values, which are accepted and understood throughout the organization. Thus, the organization should have a strong sense of mission, reflecting both a commitment to its users as valued human beings, and also a clear direction in terms of the sort of impact it sets out to have on people's lives. Many services have very clear statements of the values on which they are based and devote considerable effort to building the commitment of staff to those values. This is not easy to achieve in practice. Even where there is a written commitment to the value of clients as individuals, this may not inform the everyday practices of those who work in the service or those people who take important policy or funding decisions. A general commitment to the status of service users is no guarantee that those involved have a clear sense of direction. However, it is difficult to envisage how a service might actively pursue quality in the absence of a clear notion of what it is seeking to do for its clients!

This notion of a clear sense of direction is pursued in the third of the IDC's basic principles. It introduces the term 'accomplishment', which was first coined in this context by Thomas Gilbert (1978). Gilbert makes the point that it is important to distinguish between what people do (their behaviour) and the effects of their actions on the world (their accomplishments). Thus, in reviewing the quality of a service, it is the impact of that service on the lives of its users which is of real importance, not the process by which the service is delivered. Too many existing monitoring schemes concentrate on the process of service delivery, for example looking at numbers of clients served or bed occupancy rates, rather than the service's accomplishments in terms of client outcome. It is unusual to see services being reviewed in terms of the extent to which they enable clients to expand their social relationships or learn and effectively use new skills.

The fourth key principle from the IDC is that any system of reviewing quality should be geared for action. A common criticism of many methods of monitoring services is that they are divorced from action. Information is collected and passed 'up' the system but little if anything happens as a result of this information. The IDC was concern to devise an approach to service quality in which the process of reviewing quality is directly linked to decisions about the practical steps to be taken to improve it.

The process suggested by the IDC is somewhat analogous to the Individual Plan system which now forms the basis of much work with individual service users. It involves a group of people with a common interest in the service coming together to review its strengths and needs and on this basis to set goals for action. Meetings are held at regular intervals to review progress and agree further action goals. Whereas the individual-plan approach applies to individual service users, the 'Quality Action' approach of the IDC relates to the entire service. In this way it resembles the notion of 'Quality Circles' (see, for example, Dewar 1980) which is prevalent in certain industrial organizations and is becoming increasingly popular within the National Health Service.

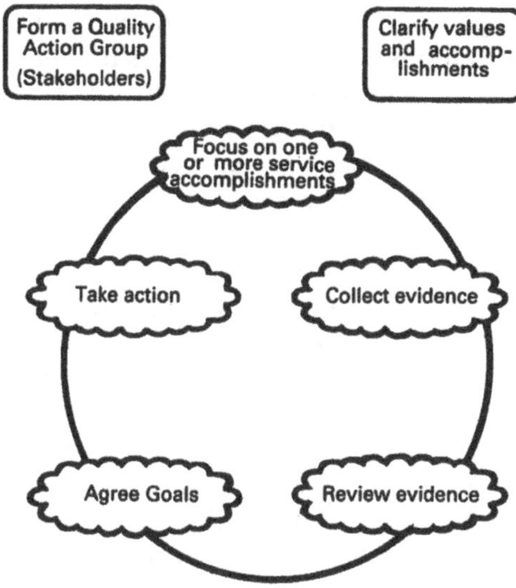

Figure 3.1 The quality action process

QUALITY ACTION: A PRACTICAL APPROACH

This approach is outlined in Figure 3.1. A working group of 'stakeholders' is formed specifically for the purpose of reviewing the service's quality and taking action to improve it. Such a group might operate at any level within a service system. It may be concerned with a particular service component (such as one residence or a domiciliary support service), a local community-based service having a number of components, or an entire service system operating over several localities.

The group first gives some attention to clarifying the values behind its service. For some services this will be simply a question of reviewing the relevant documentation and ensuring that all members of the group are familiar with this. For others, where there is no clearly stated and accepted value-base, this may be a longer process of thought and negotiation. The group also needs to consider the practical implications of these values for service users. This involves becoming clear about the service's 'accomplishments'. How does the service set out to affect its users' lives? This is a crucial step because it forms the basis of future reviews of the quality of service delivered. The group then begins a circular process. One or more of the service's accomplishments are focused upon. The group sets out to find out how successful the service is in terms of the accomplishment identified. This will involve collecting and reviewing evidence, which may come from records, conversations with users and staff, spending time in the service observing what happens, or from more formal evaluative activities, such as surveys of users.

Having collected evidence, the group reviews this specifically to determine the service's strengths and needs in terms of the accomplishment it is considering. This may well show gaps in the service or areas where improvements could be made. On this basis the group agrees goals for further action. Action may be at several levels. Thus, for example front-line staff may identify ways in which they can change their day-to-day way of working. There may be implications for staff training and a service manager may be able to take responsibility for these. High-level management or policy decisions may be needed and the group will need to identify responsibilities for negotiating these. It may not always be possible to identify appropriate action, or it may prove difficult to put this into practice because of financial or constraints. However, the group's role is to achieve what it can and to ensure that action beyond its scope is placed on the relevant agendas.

The goals set by the group should be specific and individuals given responsibility to achieve them. At a later meeting the group will review the action taken and continue the quality action cycle, perhaps moving on to a new service accomplishment.

MAINTAINING QUALITY IN PRACTICE

The procedures outlined here seem little more than common sense. It might be argued that any service with ambitions of quality should be doing something like this as a matter of course. However, from the interest shown in the IDC document and the experience obtained in trying to pilot the ideas in practice before publication, it appears that the simple notions outlined here are not a standard feature of good practice. Indeed, all of the organizations who helped with pilot work found that a considerable commitment and effort was required in order to put these sorts of activities into practice.

For many people the business of delivering services is extremely time-consuming and leaves little space for the attention to quality described above. It may not be easy to assemble a group which is representative of all the service's major stakeholders and which shares a common notion of the values underlying the service. The group's meetings need to be well planned and structured if all participants are to have the opportunity to make a useful contribution. There may be particular challenges in finding ways in which people with learning disabilities themselves can participate meaningfully in the group's work. However, experience with service organizations suggests that all these difficulties can be overcome where there is a strong commitment to the notion of pursuing quality within the service.

Ways of sustaining this effort also require some thought. It may be relatively easy to interest an organization in piloting a new approach to service quality, but what happens when the novelty wears off? Ways need to be found to ensure that the issue of quality is always high on the service organisation's agenda and that staff and others receive full recognition for their efforts in this direction. The lesson from the US commercial experience discussed above is that senior management has a major responsibility to ensure that a commitment to quality pervades the culture of the organization. How often in most service organizations do senior managers concern themselves with the details of how the service is influencing the lives of its users?

In a follow up to *In Search of Excellence* Peters and Austin (1985), in a book called *A Passion for Excellence*, discuss the practical implications for managers of adopting the management style described in the earlier book. These include the notion of 'management by wandering about', in which managers ensure that they spend time routinely with customers and with people at all levels in the organization. In services for people with learning disabilities this would involve managers ensuring that they regularly meet service users and their families and take the opportunity to talk with them about the important issues from the users' perspective. Managers might also spend time with staff and clients in various service settings. This would both sensitize them to staff issues and enable them to get some notion of how service users spend much of their lives.

Peters and Austin also discuss how managers in 'excellent' organizations take exceptional care of their customers. In our context, this would be reflected by managers showing a major commitment to the well-being of individual service users and being especially responsive to complaints or concerns expressed by them. Such managers constantly innovate. They would be concerned to try new ways of improving their service, recognizing that not all new ideas would bear fruit and learning from the experience gained.

The focus of the approach to quality action outlined here is on internal review. The group consists of people with a strong interest in the service. At some stage it will also be useful to involve outsiders in the review process. This gives fresh insights and can lead to constructive questioning of some of the ways of operating which are taken for granted. Thus, the quality action process described here can be supplemented by an annual review using outside evaluators or a facilitator from outside the service organization. Some services, for example, make a point of contracting a different form of external review each year. This may include a PASS evaluation (Wolfensberger and Glenn 1975), and contact with one of the various research groups or consultants who may be able to conduct an external evaluation or facilitate a workshop or 'programme design session' involving both staff and service users.

The early experience obtained with this approach has been primarily at the front line of service delivery. Whilst service managers have been involved, the immediate concern has been with the patterns of working of front-line staff. The IDC envisaged that its approach would equally be applied at other levels in the service organization, for example at a county or district level by the relevant managers reviewing their services' accomplishments on a broader geographical basis. The ideal would be for various interlinking quality action groups to be established, each focusing on the impact of the service on clients, but from their own perspective in the organization. A group at county level, for example, would be concerned with the broad impact of the service in terms of the numbers of clients supported in various living situations, whilst local groups would concentrate on more detailed assessment of service quality.

IN CONCLUSION

In this chapter the notion of quality in the context of services for people with learning disabilities has been examined. An important aspect of quality is the effectiveness of services, in terms of the way that they influence the lives of their users. Unlike many commercial organizations which can easily measure the quality of their products in concrete terms, it is often more difficult to define quality in terms of the impact of services on people's lives. However there is much to be said for the notion of a service organization's culture being centred around the quality of its users' lives.

The Independent Development Council's initiative 'Pursuing Quality' has been cited as one example of an approach which attempts to ensure that the issue of quality remains high on the organization's agenda. This is one way in which quality can be regularly reviewed by key stakeholders, in terms of the impact of the service on its users' lives and in ways which lead to practical improvements.

There is clearly a long way to go before services for people with learning disabilities are able uniformly to maintain quality at a high level. However the development of new initiatives along the lines set out in *An Ordinary Life* and illustrated in this volume create both the opportunity and the necessity to ensure that the issue of quality is given a high priority as new services, oriented towards improving the lives of their users, are developed.

ACKNOWLEDGEMENT

This chapter is reproduced with the kind permission of King Edward's Hospital Fund for London. It also appears as Chapter 9 in D. Towell (ed.) *An Ordinary Life in Practice*, King's Fund, London, 1988.

REFERENCES

Audit Commission (1986) *Making a Reality of Community Care*, London: HMSO.

Blunden, R. (1980) *Individual Plans for Mentally Handicapped People: A Draft Procedural Guide*, Cardiff: Mental Handicap in Wales, Applied Research Unit.

Dewar, D. L. (1980) *The Quality Circle Guide to Participation Management*, Englewood Cliffs, NJ: Prentice-Hall.

Gilbert, T. F. (1978) *Human Competence: Engineering Worthy Performance*, New York: McGraw-Hill.
Independent Development Council for People with Mental Handicap (1986) *Pursuing Quality: How Good are Your Local Services for People with Mental Handicap?*, available from IDC, 126 Albert Street, London NW1 7NF.
O'Brien, J. (1987) 'A guide to personal futures planning', in G. T. Bellamy and B Wilcox (eds) *A Comprehensive Guide to the Activities Catalog: An Alternative Curriculum for Youth and Adults with Severe Disabilities*, Baltimore, Maryland: Paul H. Brooks.
Peters, T. and Austin, N. (1985) *A Passion for Excellence: The Leadership Difference*, London: Collins.
Peters, T. J. and Waterman, R. H. (1982) *In Search of Excellence: Lessons from America's Best-run Companies*, New York: Harper & Row.
Wolfensberger, W. and Glenn, L. (1975) *Pass 3: A Method for the Quantitative Evaluation of Human Services*, Toronto: National Institute on Mental Retardation.

Chapter Four

COMMUNITY CARE

In pursuit of quality and excellence

CHRIS HEGINBOTHAM

A well-known industrialist of the 1960s was wont to say 'when you sleep on the floor you can't fall out of bed'. He was of course referring to the entrepreneurial spirit – if you have nothing to lose, whatever you try can only make you better, not worse off. And so it is with community mental health care and with community care for mentally handicapped people and confused elderly people. There is little to call a comprehensive community service – whatever we do a bit better than at present is likely to be a substantial improvement on the paucity of current care; but the analogy can be taken a step further – community care should be about the ground-floor, the grass roots, the consumer. The development of community care should seek to work from the bottom up, assessing user needs and developing services appropriately. Instead, too often, we have top-down imposed solutions to what are essentially local needs.

Community mental health care is in danger of getting a bad name, not because it has failed, but rather because it has hardly started. Detractors point to paucity of services which are under-funded and unconnected, poorly co-ordinated, patchy, and unreliable. The policy of closing hospitals has not been matched by the development of local care. Closure programmes are now coming to fruition after years of tedious planning, yet the funds to provide local services are either non-existent or too small, and the development of care is frustrated at almost every turn. Mentally ill people, mentally handicapped people, and elderly people are supposed to be the priority groups – yet that is almost a form of newspeak. Indeed, as recent debates have shown, the 'priority' groups are in danger of becoming the lowest priority of all. Many are now talking about the 'old' priority groups, the new priority being acute sector care for the seriously physically ill.

Community mental health care is much more than an alternative to hospitals. One serious problem with the Griffiths report is the misunderstanding of what a collaborative and comprehensive community care service could mean. The Audit Commission (1986) in its report *Making a Reality of Community Care* seemed to understand this point. Although deleted from the final report, the Audit Commission had stated that the danger as they saw it was moving from institutional care to residential care by-passing community care altogether. Sir Roy Griffiths's review demonstrates the failure of co-ordination: on the one hand a cheap option residential service organized by local authorities, and on the other hand a 'white coat' health service provided by health authorities.

But this is not community care. Community care demands that health, housing, social services and voluntary agencies in the private sector work together to provide a range of services, to develop choice for the user, and to meet needs in the most appropriate and relevant setting which will best help the user to re-establish the life-styles users want for themselves.

Closing the hospitals is a worthwhile aim. Every serious commentator knows that the large hospitals are no more than warehouses for the most vulnerable in society. Many of these institutions are over 100 years old, their design is outmoded, their fabric crumbling. Of course, good services can be provided in poor physical surroundings; but the very environment of these hospitals militates against good care. Corridor-like wards where thirty people live with no privacy, in conditions that the professional staff of the service would not tolerate for an instant in their own homes; this is the lot of 60,000 people, sometimes for years on end. Large institutions try – and fail – to be all things to all people. They try to be acute in-patient units, long-term care and sustenance centres, leisure, recreation and employment centres, industrial rehabilitation, day-care, housing, and residential services all rolled into one. It is not surprising that this mishmash and multiplicity of services is impossible to manage and organize properly. Patients rapidly become lost, institutionalized by a system which reduces individuality to a minimum.

There are, of course, some good large hospitals or at least parts of those hospitals; there are some good and dedicated staff working in those hospitals. But as Yeats put it:

> The best lack all conviction
> Whilst the worst are full of passionate intensity.

With a few exceptions, the best by and large lack conviction, and the worst are full of a passionate intensity to get home as soon as possible and away from the surroundings of a large institution. To those who speak with the users of such services, and help to advocate with them and on their behalf, it is a continual surprise that staff of the services can tolerate such conditions. There are still many hospitals in the United Kingdom which do not provide personalized laundry, even for underwear. Many wards have nothing but a television on twenty-four hours a day; many hospitals still have lavatories where the doors do not lock, baths with no taps, bed areas with no personal hanging space, eating areas where the stench of stale tobacco smoke hangs heavy in the air.

Community care should be much better. Sadly, apart from a few bright stars the sky is heavy with cloud. Many patients discharged from large hospitals are left in bed-and-breakfast accommodation at the seaside, pushed out after breakfast and left to wander the streets until early evening. Many eke out a miserable existence on just over £1 per day. This is not what those fighting for community care wish to see. However, such community neglect fuels the ardour of those who wish to retrench on the hospitals and gives succour to those professional staff who find it more comfortable to remain institutionalist themselves rather than face the great outdoors.

Good-quality community care comprises a range of staff and services in settings in the community which are valued by all. 'Valued' means those places that we would choose to use which support and enhance life-styles for which we all strive. Life- styles differ and in a multi-cultural and multiracial country like Britain, values differ. However, some aspects of living are held dear by all – privacy, decent accommodation, reasonable day-time activity, and sufficient income to sustain an interesting life. Services should be in such settings. Fully trained multi-disciplinary staff teams should be available in sufficient numbers to meet the specific needs of each client and to ensure that relevant services are organized and co-ordinated for that person.

The future of mental health care requires three steps: a set of principles; an understanding of the components of the service which work, i.e. the building blocks of community care; and ways and approaches to implementation. A good analogy can be taken from cookery. What is a roux, why does yeast make bread rise, what is the importance of an egg in binding the ingredients together, and so on? The building blocks are the recipe – the ingredients without which the finished meal would be meaningless; and the approaches to implementation, the cooking instructions – too cool or too hot, too little of one thing or too much of another ruins the mix.

Community care is no different. A set of principles must be established. These will include the need to treat the users of services with concern and respect at all times and to involve users in the planning, development, and management of care. Services must aim to provide relevant care, appropriate to the individual's needs, locally and accessibly. Users must have choice as far as possible of the care to be provided and treatments, care, and support should recognize the multi-factoral nature of mental health. The building blocks include models and approaches which have worked in other places. This may include any of 150 different components which have been identified. In the main, however, an approach based on community mental health centres with outreach services is to be desired. Collaboration with general practitioners, social service departments, and the voluntary sector will make a health care service more comprehensive. The cooking instructions have, however, until recently been forgotten. MIND published a set of principles in *Common Concern* in 1983, and in the same publication set out a list of building blocks for community mental health care. Subsequently, conferences and workshops have established what the components of a good service would look like on the ground. Too often, unfortunately, the 'how' of the 'what' is forgotten. Implementation of good care requires a focus on four areas of service which can be summed up in four key words – respect, competence, commitment, and evaluation.

RESPECT

Respect requires that every service should treat each user with equal concern and respect. This does not mean equal treatment. Each person is different and their needs are different. However, treating them as an equal citizen means treating their specific needs in the way that they demand or at least will tolerate, and appropriate to their very specific and individual needs. Respect means gearing services to the user rather than the producer. Respect also requires participation, which in turn demands information. Advocacy with and on behalf of users is essential to enable them to contribute to the development of care and to participate in their own care. Respect also requires that services are 'relevant' – for example, to black and ethnic minority groups or women.

The reason many of our community services are still patchy and staff still cling to the institution is producer domination. Whilst staff of the service are vitally important, they are not the reason the service is there in the first place. Although this is a simplistic truth it is so often overlooked. Sadly, many staff spend the bulk of their time in concern for the institution and for themselves rather than the user. Even the best become overwhelmed by the sheer bureaucracy of health and local authorities.

A simple addition of the total numbers of staff available to a particular population, whether currently working in institutions or in a community, demonstrates how many people it would be possible to provide care for if those staff were better deployed and organized. The sheer volume of team meetings, briefings, supervision, case conferences, travelling time, training, staff selection, and the hundred and one other things that staff have to do means that the average mental health worker is user- effective for no more than 20 per cent of his or her working week. And to be contentious many staff find that more than acceptable. Constant pressure from clients or users can be overbearing. The huge range of different people working with users at various times cannot be good economics. In any one month a person with a recurrent serious mental illness living in the community might expect to see – a community psychiatric nurse (CPN) twice, a social worker twice, an occupational therapist (let us say) four times, a home help seven times, a clinical psychologist once, a housing

Table 4.1 Balance of expenditure for mentally ill people

	1976–7	*1984–5*
Mental illness in-patients	£839.6m	900.9m
Psychiatric day patients (92%)	35.6	60.4
Mental illness out-patients	39.5	62.1
NHS total	914.7	1,023.4
NHS including overhead	986.0	1,090.9
(overhead factor)	(+7.8%)	(+6.6%)
Residential mental illness	14.5	21.0
Day Care mental illness	8.8	18.0
Social workers	2.4	4.4
(social work factor)	(10.2%)	(11.3%)
LA total	25.7	43.4
LA including overhead	31.0	52.0
(overhead factor)	(+20.7%)	(19.9%)
Total	1,017.0	1,142.9
% NHS	97.0	95.5
Total residential	922.6	985.5
% residential	90.7	86.2

Source: Audit Commission (1986).

officer from the local authority once, his or her GP twice, a residential support worker (briefly) once a day, and so on. The lack of case management and key workers exacerbates this trend.

It is only too easy to be critical. Many positive developments are taking place. Gradually, community mental health centres are being established with outreach and sustenance services. The models adopted by the Torbay and Exeter Health Districts repay examination. Housing associations, in conjunction with health authorities, and other voluntary agencies have begun to establish consortia, pulling together the finance to provide appropriate support for long-term residential care. Unfortunately, even with all agencies pulling together and trying to provide services, the mechanisms for joint planning are cumbersome and problematic. Joint consultative committees between health, housing, social services, and the voluntary sector attempt to spend a small proportion of the total available on new and innovative services. Yet the bulk of money is still consumed by large institutions. Figures provided by the Audit Commission (1986) demonstrate that 90 per cent of finance still goes into institutional care and less than 10 per cent into real community services (Table 4.1).

Nurse numbers have increased as beds have reduced. (Table 4.2) Overall, most have been deployed in institutions; but the balance – the community psychiatric nurses – have contributed a great deal to the quality of community care. Nurse numbers are still too low at less than one per occupied bed; when CPN's and management nurses are excluded the average drops to less than 0.7 per occupied bed, which with shift working gives less than two nurses for every ten patients including staff on training. It is not uncommon to have only one nurse on duty at night for twenty or more patients.

Some money has been made available for community services, largely for elderly people, through the expansion (some would say explosion) of the board-and-lodgings budget. From a base of some £40 m in 1982–3 the out-turn expenditure for 1987–8 is likely to be in the region of £600m or more (Table 4.3).

Much of this expenditure has been uncontrolled and has simply fuelled the expansion of small private agencies in an uncoordinated way. Local authorities (and to some extent health authorities) have not had the resources to monitor and supervise the standards of care in such homes, and the registration of those homes is often no more than a formality. The Wagner Committee

Table 4.2 Changes in hospital staff and patient numbers (England only, mental illness hospitals and units within other hospitals)

	Average daily occupied beds *MI*	*Nurse numbers at 30 September* *MI*
1974	89,900	42,976
1975	86,900	47,259
1976	83,800	47,617
1977	80,800	49,433
1978	78,200	49,638
1979	76,500	50,305
1980	75,200	52,577
1981	73,400	55,400
1982	71,300	56,799
1983	69,300	57,422
1984	67,000	57,555
1985	64,800	57,956

Source: Average daily occupied beds – *DHSS Statistical Bulletin* 2/86, Table 3. Nurse Numbers – *Mental Health Statistics for England 1984*, Booklet 9 Table 7, and Booklet 10 Table 7. Earlier years provided by SR2C division, DHSS. Data for 1985 are provisional.

is right to put an emphasis on the safeguarding of standards in residential care and to seek proper training of staff in these homes. Table 4.3 shows the increase in the board-and-lodgings vote. Moves by the DHSS in late 1987 to cap off these charges have met with fierce resistance. If part or all of the Griffiths report is accepted or implemented, it may mean a reduction in board-and-lodgings payments, with local authorities having to meet a proportion of the costs of residential care for any persons from their areas.

COMPETENCE

Competence means staff properly trained to provide a competent service. Services can only be fully competent if they recognize and assess fully the needs of each user, co-ordinate relevant care, and ensure that those giving that care are competent to do so. This will require multi-disciplinary teams of staff trained to undertake the

Table 4.3 Trends in social security payments

Financial year	*November 1986 prices*		
	Attendance Allowance	*Invalid Care Allowance*	*SB B&L (Independent homes)*
1976–7	309	5	–
1977–8	369	6	–
1978–9	343	7	12
1979–80	352	7	17
1980–1	350	8	26
1981–2	425	8	29
1982–3	498	10	47
1983–4	562	11	119
1984–5	629	12	218
1985–6	706	87	343
1986–7	773	100	489

Sources: Attendance Allowance and Invalid Care Allowance – 1976–7 to 1984–5 from Appropriation Accounts. 1985–6 provisional out-turn and 1986–7 published forecast (Cmnd. 9789), as supplied by DHSS.
Invalid Care Allowance for 1985–6 and 1986–7 are study-team estimates based on assumptions of 60,000 and 70,000 additional claimants due to the extension of the allowance to married women.
Supplementary Benefit, Board and Lodging (Independent Homes) – 1976–7 to 1984–5 are as provided by DHSS.
Figures for 1985–6 and 1986–7 are the study-team estimates described in Appendix D.
All figures relate to the equivalent annual cost in early December within the financial year.

tasks for which they are recruited. Training is needed in attitudes as well as techniques. Management must be local, caring, supportive, and involved – too often it is remote and bureaucratic. Future dispersed services require attention to supporting and sustaining staff working in sometimes isolated settings with only one or two colleagues.

Case management will be essential. Too often users are left to fend for themselves as they fight their way through the system; often those in severe distress are moved rapidly to an institutional environment and on discharge are rarely given more than support from a peripatetic community psychiatric nurse. As community care services develop, a range of options will become available requiring co-ordination. Case management, however, has three separate components which ought to be undertaken by three different people. Those components are:

(1) advocacy for and on behalf of the individual user;
(2) the assessment of the individual together with the co-ordination of the relevant components of service;
(3) the purchase of appropriate forms of care from private or voluntary providers.

To roll these three into one has serious dangers. The person assessing the user is not in the best position to be an advocate on behalf of that user; and although the case manager could co-ordinate care and purchase care, a conflict of interest arises. If an individual case manager is expected not only to co-ordinate relevant services, but also to get the best value for money, there will be a temptation to cut corners. Only by keeping these three functions separate with a third party advocacy agency available to each user, a case manager assessing and actively demanding and co-ordinating relevant services will the user get the best care possible. The case manager will be demanding care from perhaps a local authority whose task will be to find that care, perhaps in the private and voluntary sectors. Yet that purchasing function is kept separate from the case management function. Such an approach could be cumbersome but at local level may more likely ensure that the users real needs are met.

Case management is also different from key working. The case manager will follow a client's route through the services and attempt to co-ordinate care at the right time and in the right place.

However, at each stage another specific professional person should be attached to that user as a key worker, tracking the user and feeding back to the case manager on the user's needs and requirements. If a person is moving from one element of the service to another quite rapidly, for example on a treatment programme, the key worker will not be the same person for very long. A period in the psychiatric unit may require a key nurse for some weeks. Following a period of rehabilitation, the key worker may be a community psychiatric nurse, a home help, or even a volunteer; and that key worker could change appropriate to the seriousness of any recurrent distress felt by the user. This level of co-ordination would ensure that at local level the best skills of each individual were met in the most practical way, minimizing the horrendous waste of professional time in most services at present.

COMMITMENT

The third key word is 'commitment'. Commitment is needed from professional staff, from managers, and from politicians. Mental health care has suffered from a lack of commitment at managerial and political level. It is often said that community care does not have so much all party support as no party opposition. Community care has been building and growing for over thirty years, yet no government either of the right or the left has properly funded community services. Much rhetoric has been expended, millions of words have been written but still, forty years after the start of the NHS, community care is patchy, underfunded, and in danger of disintegration.

EVALUATION

Finally, all community services and any type of mental health care must be evaluated regularly. Every service should be reviewed and feedback mechanisms established so that staff of services know what works and what does not. One of the tragedies of the last ten years is the lack of evaluation and research into community care. The Department of Health and Social Security has been woefully inadequate in ensuring that community service developments are monitored and investigated. The only regular research co-ordinated by the department is through the Personal Social Services

Research Unit in Kent (which is looking at some thirty community care projects established out of the pile of projects programme based on the 1983 circular on 'Care in the community'), and the evaluation by GPMH (Good Practices in Mental Health) looking at some ten mental health projects. Yet this is very small beer compared to the total expenditure on mental health care, services to mentally handicapped people, and services to elderly people.

Approximately £6 billion is spent on these groups per annum. The transition from hospitals to community care is probably the biggest social upheaval of the century. It is of fundamental importance to millions of people – to those who have suffered or will suffer from mental illness, to their carers and to the community at large. Mental health care in Britain costs around £1.3 billion per annum and yet the only regular evaluation of care is done by a voluntary funded organization, the National Unit for Psychiatric Research and Development, paid for by one of the Sainsbury Trusts.

CONCLUSION

Community mental health care is at crisis point. Successive years of underfunding the health service and social services has taken its toll. Lack of planning by health authorities and local government has hindered development, as has the lack of guidance from central government. Community care cannot be a cheap option. By losing the economy scale of the large institutions, community care is bound to be more expensive. Any good staff intensive service must cost more. Mental health care has been historically underfunded and only by a significant cash injection can it be rescued. The government policy to develop community care is the right policy. The government has not recognized the cost of its own policy. Until it does so the most vulnerable people will be left with the least care.

The recently issued report by Sir Roy Griffiths offers some hope. A Minister for Community Care could give a national lead and ensure regular review of expenditure and care plans of health and local authorities. One lead agency for social care could be of great benefit, though community care is more than just social care. Packages of care tailored to individually assessed needs is an important step forward. Such packages cannot or should not be provided on the cheap. The flaw in Griffiths is to have understated the continuing co-ordination requirement between health and local authorities, particularly for mental health care.

Griffiths offers some hope, if the needs assessment and individual programme plans are properly funded, and grafted on to an improved co-ordination mechanism. More resources are essential although improved use can be made of existing staff. Setting clear objectives for each staff group and employing agency would be a step in the right direction. Whatever is done the next few years are crucial for the most disabled and frail in our society.

REFERENCE

Audit Commission (1986) *Making a Reality of Community Care*, London: HMSO

Part Two

PLANNING SERVICES

Chapter Five

DESIGNING SERVICES WITH PEOPLE WHO ARE ELDERLY

D. THOMAS, V. HOLT, M. ILLINGWORTH, N. MADDOCKS, AND E. ROBINSON

'THIS is your home now.' 'No, it isn't, I live in a house ... to make a home would need someone respectable – like you might meet at church ... who would be good and help you make your life as though it's your own again.'

'I'm not sure if I would be able to live on my own again, but dream of living in Newton Heath, in Manchester, again. I'd like people to get their act together.'

INTRODUCTION

This chapter is in two parts. The first offers some general observations about the situation of many elderly people and the serious problem we seem to have as a society in providing good-quality services. The second describes one part of a planning project which sought to involve consumers – including those with severe disabilities in designing services that might better meet their needs and begin to create a climate for radical change.

The two quotations above are extracts from lengthy conversations, observations, and analysis of the lives of just two people whom members of the project team, established early in 1986, met as part of their work. Both these women and many of the others challenged us to design and develop services which could meet their needs. They also demonstrate that it is possible, indeed essential, to involve consumers in the process of change.

The full account of this particular project – which describes both the process and a new 'home helping' model is to be found in a report entitled 'All Our Futures' obtainable from Manchester City Council (PO Box 532, Town Hall, Manchester, M60 2LA).

This report also contains a critique of sheltered housing and elderly persons' resource centres – sometimes called 'support units'.

THE EXPERIENCES OF ELDERLY PEOPLE

The first quotation is from a woman now in her eighties who has lived all her life in Ancoats, a neighbourhood close to the centre of Manchester. Having lived all her life in a home of her own – she now finds herself in an aged persons' home (APH) – just a mile away from the council maisonette from which she was admitted. Neighbours and relatives had become concerned because she was beginning to wander both at night and during the day and was no longer able to clean the house or cook for herself. However, she is now becoming increasingly sad and only smiles when she is encouraged to talk of the past, of Ancoats, of her family, and of going home. She *still* walks back in search of the house in which she grew up – long since demolished.

The second comment is from a woman who had been admitted to a long-stay hospital she had known as a child in the early 1900s as the workhouse, because she had lost the use of her legs. When the team met her, she had been there for eighteen months and her flat had been 'given up'. Whilst she did retain her dignity by creating space in an uncubicalized ward and by maintaining contact with the many friends who continued to visit her, she did not realize her dream of returning to a life in the community. She died in hospital early in 1987.

SOME MORE QUESTIONS

'What do you say – after you say goodbye?' was the attention-getting title chosen by the conference organizers – who indicated in their subtitle that they also wanted to focus on the run-down of long-stay hospitals and other institutions. It made it clear that there is an interest not *just* in systems – policies, strategies, and organizations – but in *people*. The question implied seemed to be, 'How can *human* services be made to work for people?' – or perhaps, 'Can they?'. However, this is not the only kind of question that should be asked:

Do many thousands of pensioners really need to come to live in long-stay hospitals, rest homes, nursing homes, or local authority aged person's homes in the first place?

Do we ever really say 'Hello' – especially to those with serious disabilities?

How can we begin to provide service safeguards to important *continuities* of personal identity, of place, of relationships?

How *do* you say 'Goodbye'?

How do we help service personnel to deal with the kinds of 'goodbyes' that often seem to bring with them personal criticisms – for example, when it is decided that a hospital or 'home' should close?

How do we develop strategies which allow contraction and closure to be seen in positive terms rather than as a dying enterprise?

What now seems like *thousands* of newspaper articles, television and radio programmes, official inquiries, and research reports, even before one starts to draw on personal knowledge and experience, stands as an indictment of many of our services for elderly people in a society which claims to be civilized. It testifies that much voluntary, private, and statutory care – particularly residential care – is at the best restrictive and at the worst degrading both for those who receive and those who provide it. For some it results in a premature, frightening, and lonely death.

SHARED DISABILITY

Other chapters illustrate some of the major uncertainties that exist amongst professionals as they seek to confront and perhaps find answers to questions of this find. Some moved uneasily between 'rights' as a socially defined concept which should embrace *all* citizens – including those who are elderly and have the most severe disabilities – and *needs* as an essentially professional construction that is necessarily influenced by other social and organizational values.

There seems to be an on-going struggle between optimism and pessimism. Can it be done? Can our services change? Yes, in some places this is happening. But can the more person-centred approach be sustained? (or is it just a fashion) and can it become widespread? There are also questions about technique and technology. Do we need individual care plans? Is there a need for 'case management'? How can we inspect and monitor private care? And the conversation stopper, 'but even if we want it, do the public and relatives want people with severe disabilities to remain in or return to their communities, their neighbourhoods?' Who is the consumer, anyway? In fact, it was evident from some of the discussion at the conference that 'informal carers' are seen by many as *primary* consumers!

In trying to grapple with the quagmire of doubt, it is clear that many if not most people working in human services start with a number of serious disadvantages. These include the following:

Most of us have no direct experience of being severely disabled.

Many of us do not have close unpaid personal relationships with people who have severe disabilities.

Even unpaid carers – because of the lack of support from other members of their family, from neighbours, and from the state – may have themselves come to devalue their own relatives. Even those who have not done this may have no pictures of alternative patterns of support that do *not* involve removal of the elderly person from his or her own home, neighbourhood, and community.

Many consumers and potential consumers likewise lack a vision of alternative possibilities. They cannot envisage a life with value and meaning following the occurrence or onset of serious disability. They have low expectations. They lack the information, will, and support to fight against private and public bureaucracies which themselves have become so complex that they have difficulty in allocating resources and responsibility in a coherent manner. Often the person's own sense of identity and personal worth is so affected by his or her experiences that she comes to blame herself.

A similar range of disadvantages faces human-service workers. Often those in direct personal contact have not had the space, time, supports, and settings in which they could develop good

> relationships with elderly people. Those who are most likely to be able to set and shape their organization's values are likely to be most distant from and ignorant of the day-to-day experiences of those who use services.

Paul Williams has talked about our mutual handicaps (Williams 1978). It is not just those with disabilities who become handicapped – it is also those without physical, sensory, or mental impairment. It is not just disabled people who are constrained in their experiences and opportunities, but other members of society and perhaps in particular human-service workers. Geoff Shepherd's chapter (2) refers to the need for staff to be 'liberated'.

These general attitudes pose one level of problems. In addition, there are inevitable conflicts of interest for paid workers within human services which make it difficult to continue to put the disabled person first. Beyond this, however, much of the professional training ill equips people for the job of working within and across agencies. Thus, for example, much of the work will be close within groups – some small, some large; but little of our training is directed towards understanding or being effective in such collectives, and much current general management doctrine encourages individualistic leadership.

Much of what has already been said about the failure of our services to meet the wishes and needs of the most disabled elderly would not be widely disputed. Where people differ is in the level and nature of the explanations offered. Some believe that the way forward lies in essentially structural changes within and between human-services bureaucracies. The proposals concerning changes, in agency responsibility in the Audit Commission's 1986 report *Making a Reality of Community Care* constitutes one example of such an approach.

Policies designed to increase the spread of private care are yet another example of structural or organizational changes – this time with the individual creating 'market forces' which will, it is argued, lead to improved quality of care. Yet another approach is one which seeks to reduce organization complexity and the 'remoteness' of human services by decentralizing power and resources to 'neighbourhoods'.

Another school of thought would argue that until and unless some of the higher-level values and political systems which produce and maintain prejudice are tackled, the only safeguard for severely handicapped people is likely to lie in personal relationships and commitments that are made informally outside human services.

Our view is that a combination of strategies is required. One is the one we adopted – that of making a start within existing bureaucracies so that service design and planning work is done *with* consumers *and* in a way in which commitment to change can be generated initially within the project group. It was also hoped but not subsequently realized that this kind of planning would generate commitment to inter-agency *action* beyond the project.

THE PROJECT

During 1985, concerns were being expressed in North Manchester that elderly people were having to stay in hospital long after any necessary and reasonable convalescence from illness or accidents. Some were actually living out their lives in hospital. As another speaker at the conference pointed out, this was a contradiction of concept. Hospitals are for treatment. Patients are expected to get better. This fundamental contradiction did not escape the notice of the very elderly people we met in what had become a hospital from which very few returned. However, social workers were understandably reluctant to arrange transfer to private 'rest' or 'nursing' homes and there were few vacancies in the local authority's APHs. Many were dissatisfied with the physical environment in these homes.

Whilst each agency had somewhat different expectations of the project, there was agreement that the planning of services for elderly people needs to be accorded higher priority and that a joint approach was essential. Beyond this, it was recognized that there may be merit in allowing a group of officers time out from other duties to 'think' in a considered and coherent way. (The initial title which we amended was 'THINK TANK'.)

These beginnings meant that the group had a lot of freedom to develop its objectives and methods of work. It also encouraged an interactive approach – initially with Chief and Senior Officers – which we hoped could continue as we attempted to develop our ideas and create a climate of interest and excitement. Without a wider sense of ownerships, not just for new forms of services but for a different approach to planning, we felt it was unlikely that significant change would occur in attitudes towards old people and the quality of the services.

These discussions led to a broad remit of the following kind:

> To consider and make proposals for alternatives to long-stay hospitals and Part III care, especially with regard to people with serious mental and physical handicaps.
>
> To consider the wishes and needs of the more able-bodied elderly living in the community.
>
> To make proposals regarding various aspects of housing policy for elderly people in North District.

It was agreed that the project would be most likely to succeed in furthering objectives of all three departments if it:

(a) developed ideas for services based on consumers' views, experience, and needs;
(b) made recommendations which in effect widen the options available to old people;
(c) emphasized the need for a more co-ordinated joint approach to the planning and organization of services;
(d) worked in a way which sought to promote a climate for change and to mobilise support which would enable improvements in services to take place.

It was agreed that a *shared* understanding and analysis was required as a basis for 'model building'. The background and experiences of members were very varied. Some had extensive experience of work with elderly people in one setting but not in another. Some had little direct experience with elderly people or with elderly people with serious handicaps. The team hoped to be able to offer vivid and convincing pictures of elderly people, their situation, and their hopes in a way that might generate commitment to action inside and outside the group.

The team also wanted to begin to build up a picture of major issues/questions which could be explored in other ways, i.e. surveys, general review of the literature, and visits. Out of this it was hoped to develop some service design principles with which we

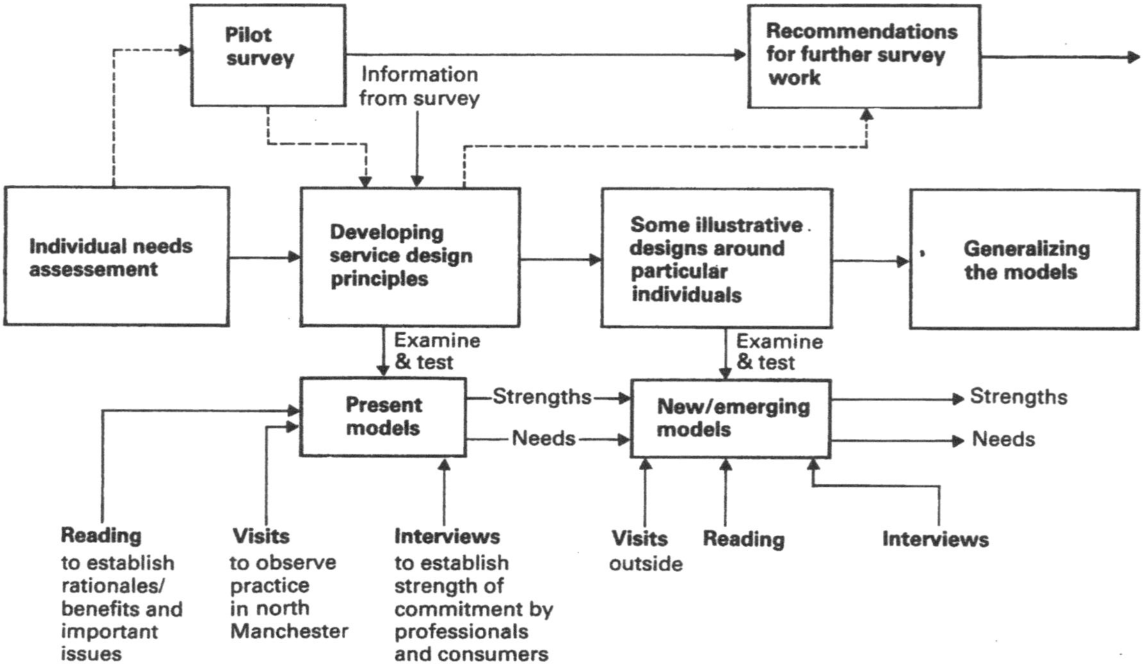

Figure 5.1 Relationship between new service design generation and collateral activities

could all associate ourselves and were grounded in what they had found about some old people they had met.

Finally, the team wanted to show that alternative models were both desirable and feasible in a way which generated a commitment action and a development strategy. Figure 5.1 shows in schematic form the relationship between the main stream of work – generating new service design around individuals – and two collateral activities, survey work, and reviewing the strengths and weakness of current and emerging service models.

The aim was to build an understanding of the lives, experiences, and wishes of elderly people for whom services were to be developed. Traditional approaches to planning can be criticized on the grounds that they represent attempts to solve (often rapidly) service problems, for example the need to replace an existing service which is being closed or run down, or that they represent the imposition of 'standard' solutions tried elsewhere. Sometimes there are pressures towards the adoption of a particular organizational arrangement. These, in turn, can lead to a preference for one service model rather than another. Here it is not uncommon for a *post hoc* philosophy to be invented to explain the choice. Alternatively, the professionals are asked to 'develop a philosophy'.

The form of service which emerges often represents a response to pressure (waiting lists, and so on) which reflects inadequacies in other services. Rarely are consumers involved or consulted. When this happens it is most likely to be a speedy response to consumer pressure 'to do something'. Rarely is there time or is time made to find out what consumers really need and want.

Another objective was to develop some understanding of the communities in North Manchester, their strengths and deficiencies and the policies which have helped to shape them, and also their traditions. In addition, there was a wish to identify key processes, for example those which occur at times of crises, which if not effectively managed may exacerbate problems and constrain rehabilitation efforts.

With regard to the central stream of work, the 'accomplishments' framework developed by John O'Brien (1987) was used as a way of generating questions for visits to individuals in their own homes, and to particular programmes (aged persons homes and the long-stay hospital). Parts of the 'Getting to know you' process developed by Marcia Brost et al. (1982) were also used to create a structure for observations, fact-finding, and conversations with individuals. Finally, the programme design techniques described by John Yates (1980) were used to examine common experience of elderly people, and to generate service design principles.

Accomplishment is the word chosen by O'Brien to describe essential life-experiences which people tend to value and to seek. They are described as accomplishments because

> they are the result of personal investment, focussed attention, and learning through action; they cannot be manufactured through a mechanical process. However, they can be nurtured and supported by other people in the way they relate to us, think about us and convey their beliefs and feelings about us to other people. They can also be encouraged or constrained by the specific human service programmes that we design and develop and can be shaped by the kind of communities to which we belong
>
> (O'Brien 1987)

At another level it is possible to ask questions about the extent to which policies and systems are likely to have positive or negative effects on the achievement of a good quality of life, by an individual. All or most of these accomplishments are likely to be those that characterize the people we tend to emulate or see as successful. Often they are missing in the lives of those with the most severe handicaps. More importantly, they are often regarded by *others* as not relevant or of less importance. Our services tend to work against their achievements by disabled people. However, those who have the most severe handicaps are most likely to need the help of others if they are to have a good quality of life and to contribute to the communities of which they are a part.

The five accomplishments identified by O'Brien are:

(1) Presence – people should continue to share their lives with other members of community.
(2) Capability – people should carry on doing things for themselves and for other people.
(3) Participation in relationships – people should have opportunity to continue with their existing relationships.

(4) Positive identity – people should have and be able to maintain their status, dignity, respect, and self-esteem.
(5) Autonomy and choice – people should retain control over important aspects of their lives.

Using these headings, the team worked to generate more specific questions.

Presence

If our services are to enable old people to continue to share their lives with other community members the following questions need to be asked.

(1) Where is the service located in relation to ordinary members of the community? Is it near to friends, informal carers, social resources? How accessible are these contacts?
(2) What happens and where during the day, evening, and at weekends.
(3) Does the service *group* elderly or impaired people together; and in what numbers?
(4) What arrangements are made to encourage positive participation with the community? Do old people get to ordinary meeting places used by other members of the community? What arrangements are made to encourage contact? Is transport adequate and available? Are there people available to accompany the old person if necessary?
(5) Do paid helpers understand the issues? Do they have a knowledge and contacts with ordinary places and people – for example, adult education?
(6) What supports or barriers does the local community offer to old people who wish to share their lives with others in the community? – for example, is there adequate street lighting, ramps, and so on?

Capability

If the service is to enable old people to carry on doing things for themselves and for other people:

(1) How are capabilities assessed? Are individual styles of coping and learning respected?
(2) How is deterioration detected? What is done about it?
(3) Are people given space and time to learn? What aids to learning are available?
(4) How does the service encourage the development of new skills?
(5) What steps have been taken to adapt the new environment? Are there adequate ramps and rails? Appropriate mobility aids? Memory aids? Aids to personal care and communication?
(6) What are the main barriers and constraints? Are the service personnel aware of them?
(7) How does the service assist people to do things they find rewarding?
(8) How does the programme encourage access to new experiences?
(9) What steps are taken to build and maintain confidence?

Participation in relationships

(1) Does the programme encourage and assist the maintenance of existing relationships?
(2) Does the programme encourage and assist the development of new relationships?
(3) What is the quality of relationships with paid carers?
(4) Are they assisted in reviewing relationships with those in their care?
(5) Are the settings ones which increase opportunities and motivation for establishing new relationships?

Positive identity

If the service is to enable old people to maintain their status, dignity, respect, and self-esteem:
(1) What images are projected about the people by the location and type of building, the signs advertising it, the language used to and about old people, the routine, rhythms, and activities of the place?
(2) Is privacy and personal space valued and if so what safeguards to this, both physical and psychological, are there?

(3) Is the importance of seeing the person in the context of their whole life recognized? Who they were, who cared for them, who they cared for, where they lived, their achievements?
(4) What roles are encouraged?
(5) What protection is offered for the person's positive identity against processes of natural ageing and/or deterioration?
(6) How does the service encourage and support the maintenance of positive identity?
(7) Does the service encourage and support positive appearance in dress, posture, hair-styles, jewellery?
(8) Are the paid helpers valued?
(9) Is the help that is offered patronizing?
(10) Is there knowledge by the staff of the personal strengths and skills of the old people?

Autonomy and choice

If their service is to enable old people to retain control over important aspects of daily living:

(1) What alternatives were available to the old person when they first asked for a service? How much time and effort was spent on seeking alternatives? How much risk is being accepted? How much pressure was on the old person to accept the service offered? Was it a crisis or a choice made over a period of time?
(2) Within the service what options are available? What choices and supports in making those choices? Is there permission to make a mess, especially where an individual is constrained through disability?
(3) What arrangements are there for money management?
(4) What arrangements are there for drug management?
(5) How does the service handle terminal care and death?
(6) What opportunities are there for old people to define and express their own needs? What do they do, when, and with whom?
(7) Do staff encourage options outside the service control?
(8) What are the expectations of users?
(9) What supports for these approaches and activities (1–8) does the system offer in planning, management, positive monitoring and evaluation, resourcing?

(10) What legislative constraints are there to autonomy?
(11) How does the service interact with the system, for example, aged persons' homes (APHs) with the social services department (SSD)?
(12) What rights are there of repeal and redress?

The framework of questions, along with some ideas from the 'Getting to know you' process, was used on several visits. There were 'team' visits organized so that a full 24-hour cycle was covered. A main purpose was to meet people who were experiencing the two forms of service for which the team had been asked to consider alternatives. Each member of the team spent time getting to know as well as possible two or three people, as well as talking briefly to others. Staff members were also asked about the people with whom they worked. Here the team wanted to know not just what they knew about a particular person, but also how they felt about old people and the work they were doing. Information was also obtained from written records; often this was very limited. This in itself was important in that it demonstrated how little importance is currently attached to the 'accomplishments' of old people, both past and present, and how easy it is for old people who are admitted to hospital or residential care to lose any sense of personal continuity.

Often, the team just sat watching and listening in dayrooms, in dormitories, in dining-rooms, in order to experience at first hand the rhythms and routines of the day, both the flat empty spells and the bustle associated with particular times of the day and routines (mealtimes, bathing, toileting). The team used the framework of questions already outlined and, in addition, looking back and to the future, asked what had life been like?; what is it like now?; what does the future hold?

Next, the team pooled observations, feelings, and ideas to produce a collective picture. In one exercise the team simply recorded all its impressions of the people that it had met and impressions of the programmes – its purposes, actions, physical environment, and so on.

The inescapable conclusions were that the rich, varied histories of these people and their contributions as workers, parents, carers, or just members of the community had been 'lost' or forgotten. Their current life-style and experience was vastly different from

Table 5.1 Themes, needs, and principles

Themes	*Needs*	*Principles*
● Lost homes and tenancies ● No security of tenure	● To stay in your own home if you wish ● To have a place that is yours with security of tenure	● Elderly people should be able to live where they choose, in a house of their choice
● Poor quality buildings ● Physically isolated	● To have a home which looks like a home (in a local neighbourhood)	● Elderly people should have available to them decent ordinary housing
● Major/multiple handicaps ● Some unable to communicate ● Little technological help	● Not to be restricted totally by handicap ● To have a home which helps you, not constricts you	● Accommodation must be designed for or adapted to individual disabilities and to changing disabilities
● Little space/privacy ● No personal possessions	● To have adequate space and privacy	● Accommodation must be available for people to move into early, at their pace ● Housing design must respect people in need for space and privacy
● Few options, little choice ● Admission sudden, chances whether you go to hospital, APH, or stay put ● Rarely a positive choice	● To have choice ● To have real choice to stay or leave	● There should be real choice available ● Services should not just come in times of crisis ● Services should support people in their choice and not give up on them
● See themselves as a burden ● Admission lifts a burden from neighbours, families, professionals	● Not to be a burden on relatives, and so on	● Informal carers should be supported, not supplanted. ● Help should be given at the consumer's pace ● Alternative paid support must be available

● Broken networks ● Bored lives, little meaningful conversation	● To have relationships protected – new relationships possible ● To be in contact with wide range of people	● Services need to recognize that old age can lead to a reduced number of relationships and promote new relationships and networks
● Don't go out much ● Don't use public transport ● People don't come in	● To get out and do ordinary things and meet people	● Service needs to ensure adequate transport available and someone to accompany if necessary to shops, post office, pubs, wash-house, and so on
● No sense of future ● Low self-esteem ● Valued previous roles ● Lost lives/histories not recorded and not known	● To have a future, to be able to talk to others about it, share hopes for it	● All people have worth. This implies recognizing the past and planning for the future
● Catastrophic loss of control	● To have control over important aspects of one's life	● Services should not erode people's control over their lives ● People should have maximum control over services

anything they had experienced before. (Most had been dislocated from their own communities and now shared their lives with people they had not previously known.) They were to a large extent seen as recipients of service rather than as people with much to give others.

If the lives of these people were once again to become valued and meaningful we had to ask what their needs were:

– if people are bored, what do they need?

– if people feel a burden, what do they need?

It was important that these statements of need were based on people that members of the team had met in North Manchester.

The themes and needs of these people were to become the foundations for all further discussions (Table 5.1). Similar frameworks and processes were then used to analyse in greater detail what was happening to particular individuals and to begin to construct a more people-centred service.

Here is one illustration. The first quotation at the beginning of the chapter is from a conversation with her. At present she is living in an APH which, as she reflects, looks like no home that she has lived in before. It is a building whose design only allows an essentially communal life-style with other very old people. 'I was not born here. I was born somewhere else (Ancoats). 'In Ancoats I had a mother and a father who passed away, and brothers and sisters; John, James, I can't remember their names, about six of them.' 'I wasn't brought up in here. I came here from friends. Home is where your mother has been and your sisters.'

She still has a picture of the future, even though she has now lost her home. 'To make a home, perhaps with someone respectable, someone you'd meet at church, who would be very good, make your life as though its your own.' She was born in 1896, one of a large family of five girls and two boys. Throughout her life her mother was to be the influential figure. She has few memories of her father who died when she was very young.

She attended a Church of England school between the ages of 6 and 14. She left school in 1910 to work at one of the local mills. The mill was owned by a firm called McConnells and was in Union Street (now Redhill Street) Ancoats, with only the streets separating it from Rochdale Canal. The building is still there, largely as it was when she started work 76 years ago. She spent at least 40 years with this same company in and around Ancoats. She retired from her work as a cleaner at around the age of 70.

As a child, the family moved only once, both houses being within a stone's throw of Butler Street, from Rolleston Street to Mercer Street. She talks of several boy-friends and of one in particular. She talks of going early to the cinema (The Empress, off London Road) and of waiting until this boy-friend arrived and then innocently joining the queue behind him, forcing him to pay the entrance fee to the cinema!

Sadly for her, her 'lad went missing' in the Great War of 1914–18. There were many other friends but she never married. She continued to live in Ancoats with her other unmarried sisters Ann and Amy, enjoying her hobbies of dancing and roller-skating at Belle Vue. She talks fondly of these times and of the warmth of the Ancoats people.

After her mother's death, and probably as a result of slum clearance, she moved with her two sisters to live in a two-storey maisonette. She remembers this as a period when she had little time for hobbies, being too busy with working and keeping a home. Whilst in the house, Mary died and Ann was admitted to hospital on a long-term ward, where she still lives on Ward 12.

Subsequently, local people and some of her relatives became concerned about her. She was beginning to wander both at night and during the day and was unable to clean the house and cook. This put pressure on the very good neighbours and caring relatives who began to find the burden of daily visits and the worry of her safety too much. Some support during the day was provided by the APH nearby and by a home help once a week.

She visited and then came to live at the APH. She regularly asks to return to her home and frequently walks back. At first she knew the address and location of her previous home but over the past twelve months has frequently mixed up her last three addresses in the Ancoats area.

She still worries about her sisters (although one has died). Occasionally she visits Ann in hospital and recognizes her instantly. She is still keen to visit and care for her sister even though Ann does not recognize her and is often abusive to her, requesting that her mother visits instead.

Table 5.2 Needs and service response

Needs	*Service Response*
A house or flat that looks something like her previous home but which can be adapted should Ann return	Housing department would have to be approached for suitable accommodation (2/3 bedroomed) after someone has talked to her about where she wishes to live and in what sort of house
Preparation and support at an early stage	A carer (woman) needs to talk to Miss W.B. about her home, what furniture is required, what decoration. This carer would work with her at the APH and 'move out' with her
She needs others – her relatives and neighbours, so that they understand and do not feel pressured	The service must accept risk-taking but but needs to plan to reduce risks
She needs to know that others are not worried about her (especially relatives)	The service may need to plan for her repeated searching for her previous home
She needs someone to cook for her and share a meal with her, also make sure nutrition is adequate	The service must plan to provide someone to share these tasks with her
She needs company during the day, to share her walks	
She needs to be busy doing her own shopping, cleaning, and so, on with support	Service must be able to include her in these activities, not to do it for her
She needs someone to get to know her well enough to tolerate her lack of verbal communication and understand her humour and eccentricities	Service must provide support people who are 'matched' to her

She is now becoming increasingly sad and only smiles when we talk of the past, of Ancoats, of her family, and of going home. She enjoys music and watching others dance. She is still physically fit, able to wash herself, dress herself, and take care of herself generally.

She pictures herself living in a house in Ancoats, being responsible for Ann, being busy helping, caring, cleaning, shopping for herself (at the APH when offered the opportunity to be busy she sees it as doing others a favour; what she really wants to do is clean her own home).

At this stage the team began to develop an individual service plan for Miss B. This service could enable her to return to Ancoats, but more importantly had it been available twelve months ago she need never have left the home she had lived in since 1963.

Table 5.2 lists *some* of the main needs that Miss B has, and the kind of responses the team would like to see from services. Now that she is living in an APH such an individual programme would be that much more difficult than if these kinds of supports had been available in the first place. Major effort would be required to secure accommodation, to work with relatives and neighbours and the staff at the APH. Miss B would need proper preparation for the move. Here there is a central role for a new kind of home-helping service – of the kind outlined in the main report. Three possibilities were considered.

(1) To employ a local woman to 'house share'. She would help to organize things for Miss B (and her sister) and do the cooking. Another local person would be needed to act as a back-up and relief for the 'live in' carer.
The house sharer would have a joint tenancy or be a lodger.
Alternatively, Miss B could be the lodger in a house in which the carer was the tenant.
The main problems we envisaged concerned security of tenure for whoever is the lodger and possible complications with regard to personal benefits.
(2) A second option would be to employ several home- helpers to work in her house from the start.
(3) The third option was a paid carer who lives locally.
She would be available during the day to provide meals, to go shopping with her.
She would work with the community to get help and support for Miss B.
Here it would be important to plan for a night carer who was known to her, should this prove necessary.

If an individualized programme of this kind were to succeed, it would require the involvement not just of the housing department or a housing association but also the general practitioner and other community health staff, supported where appropriate by members of the psychogeriatric service.

It was not suggested that these are easy or inexpensive options. However, the risks for Miss B of doing nothing are clear to see. She is likely to become more passive and less motivated to do things for herself. This, in turn, is likely to lead to a loss of important skills. There is a definite risk that she will gradually lose contact with the outside world and be forgotten. She may become not just sad but depressed. Some of the risks that were present in her life have been removed. Staff *may* be able to establish new relationships with her, but the context will never feel right. She has not adjusted. She does not want to adjust. She should not be pressured to 'settle down'. There could be a better alternative.

CONCLUDING COMMENT

Those who use human services should be involved directly and indirectly in the design and planning of those services. Tracking back and reconstructing a picture of the services that should have been made available at critical times to people who are now seriously disabled and may now not be able to articulate their views is a valuable process. The options generated using this kind of process are often not those that emerge from essentially technological approaches to planning. It is one way of bringing clarity, unanimity, and commitment to professionals who might otherwise have been misdirected by other kinds of personal and organization imperatives.

During the work the team became convinced that most service planning does not get close to consumers. At best it involves consultation after major decisions have been made. At worst it involves imposition of standard solutions as if all old people were the same and all communities similar. Often it does not even involve drawing on the available consumer-based research. There *are* ways in which more individualized design work can be done with consumers – even those who are seriously disabled. Since most professionals have little or no experience in this kind of planning, time is needed to learn and begin to put such new approaches into practice. Joint inter-agency planning, if it is to reflect consumer wishes and needs, takes time, and the ideas generated are likely seriously to challenge not only current models and practice but also emerging patterns of service. The approaches developed by the study group are recommended as a basis for much more local design and planning work within the various neighbourhoods that constitute Manchester and elsewhere.

ACKNOWLEDGEMENTS

The study team would like to thank Manchester City Council and North Manchester Health Authority for arranging the secondments, and Mark Burton for help in the use of the five accomplishments framework. We would also like to acknowledge the important role played by Community Mental Handicap Education and Research for the leadership it has shown in introducing and developing PASS and PASSING training within the UK.

REFERENCES

Audit Commissions Report (1986) *Making a Reality of Community Care*, London: HMSO.

Brost, M., Johnson, T., Wagner, L., and Deprey, R. (1982) *Getting to Know You – One Approach to Service Assessment and Planning for Individuals with Disabilities*, Madison, Wisconsin: Wisconsin Coalition for Advocacy.

Manchester City Council (1988) *All Our Futures.*

O'Brien, J. and Lyle, C. (1987) *Framework for Accomplishment – a Workshop for People Developing Better Services*, Decatur, Georgia: Responsive Systems Associates.

Williams, P. (1978) *Our Mutual Handicap*, Campaign for People with Mental Handicaps.

Yates, J. (1980) *Operational Procedures for Programme Design Sessions*, Taunton, Massachusetts: Centre for Training, Development and Renewal.

Chapter Six

COMMUNITY CARE MEANS NEVER HAVING TO SAY YOU'RE SORRY

Avoiding institutionalization in the community

MARK O'CALLAGHAN

The thrust towards 'care in the community' has led to a mixed response in terms of discharge of psychiatric patients into the community. From some hospitals this has been a trickle whilst from others it has been a flood. Some of these latter hospitals can boast of impressive reductions in in-patient numbers. Further, some of the catchment areas they serve appear to have adequate community resources in terms of day hospitals/centres and hostels as well. Much attention has focused therefore on those hospitals which do not appear to be doing enough. Pressure is being brought to bear on these to reduce their in-patient numbers and on many even to close. These in turn may complain that they are awaiting adequate resources in the community before they can discharge their patients.

There is a danger that the debate concerning 'care in the community' might just focus on money. The argument appears to run that if more patients can be dealt with in the community then resources should be switched there. The suggestion that such people may be better off in the community appears secondary. Further, the over-concern with numbers or quantitative aspects of 'care in the community' (numbers of patients discharged and numbers of hostel or day places in the community) leads to qualitative aspects being neglected.

Thus, the quality of life of ex-psychiatric hospital patients may not *have been improved* as a result of discharge into the community but may have been *worsened*. The 'benefits' to the patient of being in hospital may include three cooked meals a day, heat and lighting (without bills), people to talk to (whether staff, patients, or visitors/volunteers), trips, holidays, and events organized by the hospital, reward money in addition to 'pocket money' (many patients become financially worse off when they leave hospital), help with any difficulties they have and security. They leave all these when they go to live in the 'community' for the somewhat vague gains of 'independence' and 'de-institutionalization'. It is debatable that merely to discharge long-stay patients without thought to these considerations may worsen their quality of life rather than improve it.

One of these ex-psychiatric patients writing in the Middlewood Centre Magazine (1984) after being discharged into the community from Solihull Social Services Rehabilitation Hostel, Middlewood House, noted:

> The main thing about leaving Middlewood and living on your own in the community is that you become quite lonesome. You can always have company 24 hours a day at Middlewood but in your own flat it is like [*sic*] living on the moon. The loneliness effects [*sic*] everyone, it must do, for the so-called 'normal people', with such a bad memory and a disabled person such as I am classified. You have nobody to talk to for most of the day and life can sometimes feel meaningless... Some of the good things are that you can please yourself on what time you wish to get up or go to bed., [*sic*] what you wish to eat or drink and when you feel like it [*sic*]. In other words you are your own boss and an independent person living in *your own* [*sic*] flat and not in a hostel.
>
> I still stress that doctors haven't yet found a cure for loneliness, a shame but there you are, that's life.
>
> (p. 10, original emphasis)

Such people like that writer are *comparatively* lucky for he still has the hostel and attached day-centre for support and company. There are many for whom 'care in the community' means being 'dumped' in the community without proper preparation and without support. Indeed, if any patients are considered at all 'difficult' then various strategies may be employed to keep them at arm's length from the institution:

(1) Discharging them into another hospital's catchment area so that after a short period of time (for example, one month)

they become the 'responsibility' of the other hospital. Continuity of care is therefore lost.

(2) Sometimes hospitals have a 'blacklist' of patients who are not to be admitted, or if so, only after a great deal of difficulty.

(3) transferring their 'care' to Social Services by suggesting that the individual does not need hospital care but still needs residential accommodation when this may not be the most appropriate place.

(4) Transferring their 'care' to their families or lodgings who may not be in the best position to care without a great deal of support which may not be provided.

(5) In some cases the 'institution' travels out to the individual in order to keep him/her in the community. Thus, Hospital Social Workers and Community Nurses pay fleeting visits to a Group Home more as a 'trouble-shooter', i.e. just to make sure that the residents are 'behaving' themselves.

(6) Arranging for them to attend somewhere else during the day and live in lodgings (some like psychiatric ghettoes). This is just to keep them occupied in sorting screws in so called 'industrial units' or sitting in a lounge with the television or making baskets in a day centre/hospital.

(7) Redefining the 'problem' as 'untreatable' or one of a social nature or one for the legal service.

These practices are not usually carried out through malice but rather through misguidance, ignorance, and inability to cope. Hospital staff themselves often feel under pressure to discharge and therefore feel that they have to keep people in the community without the proper community resources being available.

Clearly, adequate community resources are needed to avoid some of the worst excesses of community care such as appears to have happened in Italy. If not then the effect might be one of persuading some that such a 'liberal' policy cannot work and therefore risk 'throwing the baby out with the bath water'. Unfortunately, in an effort to try to get adequate provision of community facilities, much attention has focused on numbers of day or hostel places. Guidelines, as issued in the DHSS's document *Better Services for the Mentally Ill* (1975), are often seen as the goal of 'care in the community'. It is the attention to such 'bricks and mortar' issues that has led to local planners failing to consider what their overall purpose was to have been in the first place. Such facilities were meant to provide a more appropriate environment for these ex-patients in order to avoid the worst aspects of the old psychiatric institutions. Unfortunately, many of them have repeated the mistakes of the large hospitals and have merely shifted 'institutionalization' into the community.

When setting up community facilities, six issues need to be considered and therefore the rest of this chapter will go into them in some detail. However, it must be stressed that the points raised are only a personal view, often learned from my own mistakes as well as learning from the experience of others.

GUIDING PRINCIPLES

The guiding principles underlying a service need to be clearly stated. Often this is not done, which can lead to misunderstandings and difficulties during the operation of projects. Some thoughts under this rubric are set out below.

(1) Treat people as independent ('normal') as possible, i.e. like everyone else given any difficulties they may have. This does not mean putting people into situations which, although 'normal', will cause them difficulties with which they may not be able to cope. People are often returned to the very circumstances which may have led them to come into the hospital in the first place.
(2) Minimum appropriate intervention consistent with being in the community rather than 'take- over'/institutionalize their lives.
(3) 'User-orientated', i.e. services matched to the people served rather than the other way around.
(4) Focus not just on the individual but see them in the context of their family, social, and cultural circumstances – if change is needed, then these may have to be modified rather than just altering the individual.
(5) Do not patch it up – try to deal with the underlying causes of difficulties rather than just their surface manifestations.
(6) Teach strategies not just techniques, so that the individual can learn to deal with a wider range of circumstances and have wider choices.

(7) 'Natural' consequences as far as possible rather than artificial rewards or punishments.
(8) Multi-(Inter-)disciplinary co-operation rather than professional or agency protectionalism and rivalry.
(9) Efficiency so that the best service is given with the resources available but not 'low-cost' (i.e. just to save money to the detriment of the quality of the service).
(10) Continuous evaluation of the service to make sure it is meeting the needs of the population served.

COMMUNITY FACILITIES

The past few years have witnessed the establishment of a number of hostels, ranging from short-stay 'crisis intervention' centres, through medium-stay rehabilitation hostels to long-term homes. Unfortunately, whilst much time and effort has been brought to bear on finding the money (both capital and, even more difficult, the revenue costs) for such places, little considered-thought has been given over to proper planning (whether of the building itself or how it is to be run). In setting up such hostels it is sad to see planners repeat the mistakes of the old institutions; often some of the worst excesses appear to have been committed with the very best of intentions.

When establishing facilities, therefore, the following thoughts might prove useful in avoiding some of these difficulties:

(1) Is the facility *really* needed? Sometimes a facility is established because it conforms to some guideline or other such as the DHSS's (1975) document *Better Services for the Mentally Ill* which recommends that for every 1,000 population there should be *x* number of places in a particular facility. As Cochrane (1983) has shown, there are different rates of mental health problems associated with different populations and therefore different areas. Facilities should be matched to the needs of these differing populations. In a 'formula approach' one would assess the type of population to be served as well as the current use of services and then work out what facility would be needed. Thus, for example, in our own case we might require a different type of day facility in the more rural Solihull part of our catchment area where it appears that a greater number of middle-aged separated women

use our hospital services than in the inner-city Birmingham part where single men in their early thirties are more represented.

(2) As well as being appropriate to the population served the facility should be capable of matching any individual user's special needs (for example should cater for physically handicapped people). In our own case our two rehabilitation hostels can accommodate physically handicapped people whilst our main hospital rehabilitation unit cannot.

(3) If we are going to avoid one of the major errors of the past, then we should ensure that the facility is within the community it will serve, with easy access to it, rather than being stuck on the periphery of the area or outside it. In our own case our two rehabilitation hostels are located within the respective communities they serve and have good access by public transport (used by most of our 'consumers') our main hospital rehabilitation unit lies some 12 miles away from the *nearest* part of our catchment area. A large Social Services day centre lies on the very outskirts of Birmingham with poor public transport access to it, providing the only Social Services mental health day centre for approximately one million people.

(4) To prevent 'attitudinal' as well as 'geographical' isolation it is essential that the facility should look as 'normal' as possible and therefore blend into the surrounding community in terms of the following:

(a) The same style as property around it. A large new building surrounded by ordinary housing may not be the most appropriate method of 'community care'. Some facilities (for example, Oakley House, Coventry Social Services/Church Housing Association Rehabilitation Hostel) have been built at the same time and in the same style as other surrounding houses).

(b) Conversion of existing property might in some circumstances be a more appropriate solution (for example, Flint Green, Birmingham Social Services/COPEC Rehabilitation Hostel). One must, however, be wary of its previous use (for example, one facility for elderly people was previously a *workhouse*.)

(c) Its size should be as small as possible to avoid the feeling of warehousing of individuals as well as being more like a real 'home'. This obviously interacts with economic aspects in terms of building and running costs.

(d) How the facility is 'advertised' is important in reducing 'attitudinal isolation'. Thus, for example, signs such as 'Hostel for the Recovering Mentally Ill' should be avoided. Whilst it may appear sound argument to be 'open' about mental illness, residents may suffer as a result of being ostracized by the community. For a hostel room numbers can be used and the building receive the same name as other buildings around it (for example, 6, Middlewood House, Larch Croft – a room in a rehabilitation hostel – is a similar address to 6, Woodbrooke House, Larch Croft – a flat in a nearby tower block).

(e) Fencing around the facility should be avoided or at least be as inconspicuous or similar to nearby buildings as possible. Putting up a high fence around a hostel (even in its construction stage) to keep vandals out may be construed by neighbours as being needed to keep in 'dangerous mental patients'.

(5) The design within the building is equally as important as its exterior in avoiding some of the worst excesses of the old 'institutions'. There are a number of ways in which the design buildings, even though they may be within the community, can still reflect these old institutions in a numbers of ways:

(a) Like the old institutions there is often a lack of flexibility in building design leading to the user being forced to fit to the building rather than the other way. Thus, one finds:

- Facilities (particularly the structured 'stepping-stones' units) where so-called 'bed-block' occurs whereby an individual is unable to move to another unit which is more appropriate to his or her needs because of lack of places and therefore must remain where they are at an inappropriate level of functioning. A building should be flexible enough to allow rooms to change function to suit the individual. Thus, for example, rooms in a rehabilitation hostel should be designed so that they *could* be used either as an ordinary bedroom or as a bedsit, as at Flint Green House in Birmingham.
- Similarly, buildings should be designed so that change of use could occur should circumstances arise. Middlewood

House was originally built with six places forming a group training unit for people who might go into a 'Group Home'. Since very few of our residents ever wanted to go into this form of accommodation, this led to many people being forced into living as a group whilst waiting for a place in one of the 'bedsits'. Conversion of such rooms into bedsits has eased the 'bed-block' problem.

- There may even have to be some method of meeting an individual's changing needs within the same room. Thus, for example, whilst it is a laudable aim to ensure that each resident of a rehabilitation hostel has his or her own room, some people might find that too threatening at first. Thus, for example, people coming to a rehabilitation hostel from a long spell in a long-stay ward might be used to sleeping in a large dormitory and may be anxious about sleeping in a room by themselves in a hostel which has all single rooms. Similarly, a resident may have spent all his or her life sleeping at home in a room with a brother or sister. A double room which has a movable partition in it, which can be gradually slid across as a divider as fears about sleeping alone subside, may be used to some benefit. Such an arrangement would avoid the trap of having to have a 'fixed' double room either empty or used inappropriately for single people who did not have this special need. The room could also be used for a couple since even couples require rehabilitation from time to time.
- Allied to this is the overall changing needs of the users. Facilities should be adapted to meet these needs. Thus, at Middlewood House we noted that residents no longer required meals to be provided to them but needed help in learning how to cook for themselves. The large institutional kitchen with the big hospital-type gas cooking range had to be converted to three training areas (one electric and two gas domestic cookers) in the one kitchen so that a domestic supervisor could oversee three trainees if necessary.
- Thought should be given to the resident's eventual placement and the role of a hostel in acting as a stage towards that. Thus, sufficient storage space should be allowed in hostels for residents to store their goods since

many may have their own furniture or be collecting it during their stay. It may even be appropriate to store the *hostel* furniture and allow the individual to have his or her own possessions in his or her room. Thus, the move from hostel to the community will not appear such a great step as they would be used to using their own equipment.

- Many mental health facilities cannot cater for an individual's special needs so that physically disabled people are excluded from them, thus compounding their already existing disadvantages. Establishments taking the physically disabled may not be keen to take people with mental health problems. Thus, people with such problems and with physical handicap are often excluded from facilities because these are not designed to take into account multiple handicap.

(b) The process of 'attitudinal isolation' is often found within community units. People who use the service are segregated from the more 'normal' people, i.e. the staff who have their own 'territory' which is restricted to the users. This is expressed in a variety of ways:

- separate entrance for staff and users (and even for goods!) can be found in some community facilities;
- staff have separate toilets in some places (almost as if mental illness could be caught from lavatory seats);
- 'bolt holes' are often provided which are absolutely forbidden to users where staff can 'escape' and hide from users (residents or day attenders);
- separate offices are a feature of establishments where staff themselves are segregated into 'senior(s)' and 'juniors', the 'chief' having a separate office from his or her 'junior' staff;
- specialist rooms, particularly in day units, also serve to divide staff where different professionals regard having a separate office as a mark of professionalism. In extreme cases a room will be designated for a particular purpose which, whilst only required for a short period each day, will be excluded to others users (for example, a specialised art-therapy room).

(c) In many community facilities, users are even segregated amongst themselves, particularly on sex lines. Like children, they are regarded as being unable to cope/deal adequately with emotions, especially those involving sexual relationships. The solution is usually to separate the sexes in terms of:
  - their bedrooms (and, in some establishments, even sitting-rooms) being separated into separate 'wings'.
  - monitors (for example, electronic switches tripping off lights on a control panel) are used in other buildings where there are not separate wings but staff still wish to see who is entering whose room;
  - toilet facilities even in buildings professing to be 'like home' are separate for the sexes, unlike a really normal home.

(6) The fabric of a building can give it the stamp of an 'institution' in a number of ways:

(a) 'Public' buildings will clearly be subject to more use than private homes and therefore for economy's sake fabric used in the unit may need to be hard-wearing as well as easy to maintain whilst still retaining a 'normal' appearance.
(b) Related to this is that many facilities have fabric which can only be cleaned by special equipment (for example, special floors) rather than by the clients in rehabilitation hostels.
(c) Special needs must be catered for so that, for example, non-slip flooring may have to be installed in kitchens where clients (for example, the elderly) may have difficulty in walking, especially if the floor gets wet.
(d) In rehabilitation and longer-stay hostels, in particular, the 'personal touch' should be encouraged wherever possible. Thus, clients should be allowed to paint their own rooms and have their own displays, subject to similar sorts of regulations as ordinary council house tenants.

(7) Almost above all else the fittings of an establishment can give it the air of 'the institution' (especially if they are large and 'antiseptic'). The following may need to be considered:

(a) 'Industrial units' for the sake of economy rather than appropriateness in places designed to teach people how to live independently such as in rehabilitation hostels. These include:

- Large cooking ranges instead of ordinary domestic cookers (or even 'Baby Bellings' for those going into bed- sits). It must be noted here that both gas and electric cookers for training should be provided since some clients will be going to places where gas might be supplied and others where electricity is the sole form of power.
- Deep freezers to store large joints of meat and bulk packages of frozen food rather than ordinary fridges (or even small fridges to store food for one person going into bed- sits).
- Large pantries/larders to store bulk provisions instead of small cupboards to keep a week's shopping for one person.
- Dishwashers are often supplied which reflect the 'rota' method of rehabilitation whereby one person cooks for *x* number of people every *y* numbers of days with another doing the washing up. The dishwasher is therefore 'needed' for the large amount of washing up. Instead, people should be taught to cook for themselves if they are going to live on their own and therefore wash up for themselves as well.
- Launderette facilities are provided which are not realistic. If there is no access to a launderette in the community then the individual should be taught how to wash by hand or use a domestic washing-machine if they are likely to get one. Unfortunately, in many hostels a 'launderette' is provided on site in which clients can wash one article of clothing in a large machine full of washing powder. Economy is not taught as part of this training for it is hoped (if it is even thought about) that the individual will learn all about that once discharged.

(b) Unfortunately, many of the more institutionalized aspects of these buildings come from 'official requirements' which are designed for 'public buildings' rather than for ordinary homes as in the following:

- 'Health and Safety' places many restrictions in the kitchen which would not be seen at home. Whilst some are welcome, others appear incongruous, such as an extra handbasin in the kitchen, something which does not occur in ordinary homes.

- Fire regulations festoon such places with fire doors, smoke detectors, fire panels, and warning signs. Unfortunately, these can ruin a homely atmosphere and therefore when designing a new building or converting existing premises, care should be taken to minimize the fire risk and thereby avoid the need for such items.
- Other regulations may come about through Registration of Homes or local authority (or similar bodies') requirements.

(c) Further, care must be taken to cope for the 'non standard individual'. Whilst this might include those with special needs such as physically disabled people, it ought to take into account non-standard 'Dwarfs' and 'Giants', i.e. smaller and taller people. One hostel, for example, had cupboards fitted high up on walls which people under five foot two inches could not reach easily and plugs which were so low that people over five foot ten had difficulty in using.

(d) Finally, one must be careful of regarding some fittings as reflecting institutionalized attitudes when they may sometimes be appropriate, as in the following examples:

- In some facilities one notes that staff have their own jealously guarded cups or mugs which clients are not allowed to use. Such practices can further alienate staff from residents. However, in some hostels staff have their own cups since the practice is that residents have their own crockery for which they are responsible and which is used in their training and which they might even take with them.
- In some hostels, paper-towel dispensers rather than ordinary towels are fitted in toilets. This may well be inappropriate in those facilities shared by few people (for example, where four bed-sits are grouped together), but in toilets used by many (including both day-attenders and staff) it may be more practical and hygienic.

STAFFING

The staffing of community facilities comprises the largest element of running costs. There are quantitative and qualitative aspects to staffing.

Quantitative Aspects

Here one is considering the number of staff, or perhaps more appropriately staff hours, since one is more concerned about having staff deployed at appropriate times rather than just a number of bodies. There are a number of considerations to be borne in mind when fixing staff levels.

(a) First of all, should guidelines or formulae be used in assessing numbers? The West Midlands Regional Health Authority Rehabilitation Survey Team (1979), for example, suggests ratios of so many staff to so many patients. Such a blanket statement ignores the needs of the clients and also factors such as sickness, annual leave, and so on. A better method is the 'formulae' approach adopted by the Working Party of the Social Services Liaison Group (1978) report on behalf of the British Association of Social Workers which takes into account the issues to some extent. Thus, for example, for a hostel of mentally ill individuals of twenty-five places they recommend eight staff derived in the following manner.

Given that some individuals might require more care/training/attention (i.e. they might be more disturbed or require more help with self-care tasks or training), then the ratio would be increased to, say, forty-five, thus resulting in ten staff being needed.

(b) Planning of rehabilitation programmes should be carried out on the basis of a minimum and not an average staffing complement otherwise certain of them will have to be abandoned. In rehabilitation, consistency of programmes is crucial. Therefore, considerations of staffing should take into account as far as possible exigencies of the service so that the staffing set will be maintained and programmes will continue to run. Thus, built into staffing will be a certain amount of 'slack' which can be used to run extra short-term or on-off programmes or be used for projects.

(c) Real and not 'paper' staffing is required in that sometimes an establishment is supposed to have a certain number of staff but the actual numbers available for duty is always one less because, for example, someone is always off on a course. Thus, when establishing staffing levels, calculate the number of staff required 'on the ground' and then add extra numbers for those who will be off on courses, and so on.

(d) Staff should be employed at appropriate times. Thus, in a rehabilitation hostel where all the residents go out to work or to a day-centre, few staff need to be employed during the day at the hostel; rather they should work in the morning or in the evening when training in independence skills is required. A further important point is that at present in many residential establishments 'day' staff are employed until 8.00 pm, when night cover takes over. Similarly, a skeleton staff is employed at weekends; the argument being that nothing much goes on at these 'quiet times'. I would argue that these are the most crucial periods in rehabilitation. These are the times when social skills and leisure *training* (and not just *occupying*) should take place. These are too often the skills that are deficient in our clients when they live in the community.

Similarly, with day-centres staff are employed on a nine-to-five basis during weekdays when the real need for the service may lie outside these times, i.e. in the early evening and at weekends. However, one must avoid the danger that part-time staff are employed in the morning and other part-timers in the evening, thus losing the continuity of rehabilitation.

(e) Whilst 'booking-off' most frequently occurs in psychiatric hospitals, similar practices can occur in other 'community' settings such as in hostels or day-centres. Rehabilitation is often seen as 'icing on the cake', i.e. not part of a basic service, and therefore when staff are required by another hard-pressed unit, rehabilitation staff are taken off. The attitude taken is one of 'Well, its only Social Skills Training that's being disrupted'. However, the continuity demanded by rehabilitation is broken. It is pointless starting rehabilitation programmes which are continually going to be broken off.

(f) A similar issue is 'rotation' of staff. This usually affects psychiatric hospitals and involves moving staff who have been on a unit for a period of time to another unit to prevent them from becoming 'institutionalized'. At its most extreme (as has happened with our own service) such moves have been carried out by senior management at very short notice, with little or no real consultation with the unit involved and against the wishes of the individuals concerned. This short-sighted measure was started as a reaction to the finding in psychiatric hospitals undergoing enquiry that poor practices were being carried out by staff who had been on a particular unit for a long period of time. Thus, staff are 'rotated' to another unit to prevent institutionalization. If only it were so simple to prevent institutionalization in this way we might also 'rotate' our patients in similar fashion! Rotation is perhaps a slip-shod way of dealing with staff; it is no substitute for proper staff appraisal and management. In rehabilitation we should try to prevent institutionalization by identifying the strengths, weaknesses, and thereby needs (as well as wishes) of our staff and clients. We then try to play particular courses of action with them to achieve the appropriate goals.

(g) It is worrying that students/learners are often counted as 'real' staff. It is assumed that they are able to do the work of qualified staff. In some authorities lip-service is paid to the fact that they are supposed to be training and yet in practice they are often used as an ordinary pair of hands. If training is carried out properly then as well as adding to the service in terms of time, students/learners will also take from it because they do require teaching as well as counselling in their work.

(h) Finally, when considering staffing levels it can be useful to consider a 'resource pool' whereby instead of thinking of staff being just for a particular unit one might think of them being part of a whole service. Thus, for example, if one wants to set up a social skills training group it might be useful to have a member of the residential staff running the group with a member of the day staff. The benefits of such a scheme might include continuity of programme from day to evening and weekend. Secondly, it might encourage greater co-operation between two sections of the service (often poorly co-ordinated and sometimes at loggerheads). Further, when staff are off on holiday or ill then someone else can run the group.

Qualitative aspects

Qualitative aspects of staffing are frequently ignored or underplayed once the quantitative side has been resolved. However, they are a crucial issue in rehabilitation for the attitude as well as the skill of staff can either make or break a good rehabilitation system. Various issues need to be considered.

(a) A mixture of 'trained' and 'untrained' staff may be seen to be useful in a community mental health facility. There is little appropriate training in this form of work and therefore one usually employs staff who are already trained in a relevant profession and then hope that they can function appropriately. Thus, trained staff are usually nurses or social workers and occasionally teachers. Such staff can be useful in that they are usually not afraid to deal with any difficulties which may be encountered. However, there is the danger that they may 'professionalize' the person they are meant to be helping. Untrained staff, on the other hand, will be more likely to react to an individual 'normally' but may need help in understanding the resident or day attender. A mixture of staff in hostels can provide a stimulating environment in which there is appropriate knowledge and attitude.

(b) Irrespective of whether staff are trained or untrained it is essential that they are appropriately 'community orientated'. Thus, in their dealings with the residents or attenders they should try to ensure that what they do is appropriate to what would happen in the community.

(c) There are other attitudes which should be 'appropriate' as well. Thus, it is important that the work carried out by a member of staff should be appropriate to what would be expected in the community (i.e. as 'normal' as possible) but should also take into account the individual's level of functioning. For some individuals coming into, say, a rehabilitation hostel after many years staff may have to do more for them and provide greater supervision whereas for someone coming straight from living independently in the community such restrictions should be minimal. There are questionnaires which help investigate 'appropriate' attitudes towards rehabilitation and community care.

(d) If staff are to come on to the unit then they should be selected appropriately rather than just moved on to the unit. Selection should look at the individual's skills, attitudes, experience, capacity to learn, how he or she gets on with other staff and also with clients, patience, and consistency.

(e) Even if staff are selected appropriately then some thought must be given to ongoing training. This may have to take place at the very start of their engagement and may have to include a knowledge of the client group, techniques, and strategies of rehabilitation and community care as well as the system in which they will be working. It is important that such training be practically orientated rather than just theoretical, as in our own Rehabilitation and Community Care course.

(f) It is most useful if staff can have experience of systems other than their own. These should include those which interact with the establishment in which they themselves work. This can be done by interchanges such as we carry out in our own system. Thus, residential social workers work on a hospital rehabilitation ward for three weeks and vice versa. Similarly, it is also arranged for residential social workers to spend some time at other rehabilitation hostels within the area. Short visits can be a useful supplement to these placements.

(g) Finally, such establishments should have access to multi- (or preferably 'inter-', since this actually implies co-operation) disciplinary support. All too often community facilities are just left 'to get on with it', which they do in order to prove that they can cope. When they get into difficulties and require assistance then other disciplines can look down on them. These latter staff can also leave their colleagues with the impression that they do not think that 'community care' is working. (Re-)habilitation and continuing community support should be seen as a partnership between a number of different people including the direct care-staff, care professionals and other agencies, 'informal' carers (including landladies/lords, relatives, friends, and neighbours), and, of course, the individual him/herself.

MANAGEMENT AND ADMINISTRATION

In establishing community facilities much time is spent on 'bricks and mortar' issues, i.e. in getting the buildings and the staff, whilst little thought is given to how the place is run. In visiting hostels and day-centres in the community, one often notices an 'institutionalized' practice which on further enquiry may not be due to an individual staff member's attitude but due rather to the way the centre is run. Thus, although one may have appointed staff with appropriate attitudes and experience they are constrained to adopt institutionalized practices by their management. The chief concern seems to be making sure that it is run according to Social/Voluntary Services administration policies. Few of the directives sent from headquarters appear to have anything to do with the overall purpose of the establishment, namely the training/care of the individuals. Indeed, it may sometimes appear that the official communications are in direct conflict with appropriate practices.

The reason for this state of affairs is often quite simple. Rarely have people sat down and considered the overall philosophy of an establishment and what its aims and objectives should be and what practices should be adopted to meet them. Staff are appointed and it is assumed that they should be able to 'get on with it'. In the absence of this overall plan, staff have to look elsewhere for guidance. Thus, they adopt practices which are fundamentally 'conservative' i.e. which aim to avoid getting themselves into trouble. The outcome of these is that staff exercise a great deal of control over their 'charges' lives, i.e. in direct antithesis to independence training, in which the client is given as much freedom as possible. These practices appear in a number of ways.

(1) The first set of practices adopted can be called 'traditional' in that the staff have been used to carrying them out or seeing them carried out elsewhere. In some hostels residents are forced to have a bath and their possessions catalogued and even taken off them 'for safe keeping' on admission.

(2) A similar set of practices is due to administrative convenience. Thus, for example, money (including their own benefits) may be taken off residents and then doled out to them to suit the administration at 'Central Office'. Computerization and the use of expensive security firms has further increased this trend towards greater bureaucracy. This process of stripping the individuals of their personal responsibility and individuality is extended in many hostels by forcing them to get up and go to bed at times convenient for the staff.

(3) Some practices involved in rehabilitation hostels may include protecting clients from harm by not allowing them to manage their own medication, not allowing them sharp objects (such as razors or bread knives) unsupervised. Matches may be banned or residents not allowed to smoke in their own rooms or cook

unsupervised in case of fire or scalding. Now, whilst these 'precautions' may appear to be sensible one must consider what the overall function of the rehabilitation hostel is, and that the residents may leave the hostel and go into a bed-sit where they may smoke and cook. They should be taught *how* to smoke appropriately in the training facility rather than just be banned.

(4) Similarly, residents are not allowed to stay out late nor to have visitors except at severely restricted hours. They may also have to get up at fixed times (especially to fit in with staff shift-patterns), even at the weekends. Such practices are similar to restrictions imposed upon children intended 'for their own good'. Thus, alcohol is banned in many hostels and centres without residents being taught how to use it appropriately. Close relationships may also be discouraged (under the pretext that clients will be 'moving on'). Sexual expression is denied to many clients either through banning the sexes from meeting or through the way the facility is designed. (It is interesting to note how often inappropriate sexual behaviour is a result of legitimate sexual expression being suppressed by 'management').

(5) This lack of personal responsibility is extended so that in many establishments residents have little or no part in the planning of their own lives. Goals are set for residents and few are allowed into their own case reviews (if they are held) and they have no access to their own records so that information may be written down without them having any chance to query it.

(6) One often notes residents receiving 'block treatment'. This occurs particularly at day-centres/hospitals where residents are expected to attend all groups every weekday (irrespective of need) and at times suited to ambulance or other provided transport. It is no wonder that the average daily absence rate at day-centres and day hospitals currently runs at about 50 per cent. Such problems are compounded by practices such as timetables having seen set many years ago and then not changed to suit the clients needs.

(7) In some cases practices are described as 'therapeutic' when more careful investigation reveals that they are merely 'time-fillers'. Industrial or occupational therapy practices in particular can fall into this trap. In other instances, 'work' is provided which consists of sorting screws for 50 pence to £4 a week in a Victorian-type factory for many years with no canteen facilities

being provided. The claim that such 'work' provided by voluntary '*industrial* therapy associations' is therapeutic is belied by the fact that such 'trainees' are not reviewed (even their medication, despite some places having nursing staff assigned to them). It is interesting to note that in certain establishments which use 'contract' work to fuel 'therapeutic' activity, one notes how much the fulfilling of the contract has taken precedence over the 'therapeutic side'. Thus, for example, staff may spend a fair amount of time at certain periods actually doing the work themselves rather than training/supervising in order to finish the contract before the deadline.

(8) Financial considerations may play an important part in practices adopted by some establishments. In some residential homes or hostels, residents are required to leave the place and be out of the building between certain times. This, it may be alleged, is to encourage them to look for work or to 'use community facilities', or even 'to prevent institutionalization'. In some cases it is just a squalid attempt to save money by saving on heating and even staff costs.

(9) A related issue is that there are often pressures (inextricably linking financial and political considerations) upon such community resources from outside the facility. For Social Services establishments there is the danger of such places merely becoming 'sausage factories', turning over large numbers of clients merely to maintain high 'throughput' statistics. The consequences of such practices in terms of re-admissions and breakdowns are ignored or not even noticed (except by the local hospital). For the voluntary sector one sees the pressure to keep high occupancy-levels, which tend to keep people at a place for a long time so that revenue is not lost. Sometimes residents are kept because they are deemed to be useful, doing various jobs around the hostel. If they were to leave, another resident would have to be trained in his or her place. In other cases they are kept because they are quiet and staff do not wish to have someone else in their stead who might not be so easy to deal with.

(10) A final category of practice can only be described under a heading of 'It seemed like a good idea at the time'. Thus, a Voluntary or Social Service hostel may invite various people who provide services in the community to visit clients at the hostel or

day-centre. Special discount rates or treatment may thereby be obtained. Thus, for example, hairdressers may do a 'Tuesday' at the hostel. Residents should be encouraged and (if appropriate) trained to use as many facilities in the community in as normal a way as possible. Community psychiatric nurses and psychiatrists may hold sessions at such hostels, thereby turning then (at least in the residents' eyes) into annexes of the hospital.

One must beware of making sweeping pronouncements on practices in community facilities without careful consideration. Certain so-called restrictive practices may be appropriate for certain clients at particular stages of their training. The way a place is managed should be matched to the clients' needs rather than the other way around. Thus, a resident at a hostel may have just come from a spell of many years at a hospital. It may be inappropriate to give this resident complete control of a complex regime of his or her own medication if residents were used to having it given to them by nursing staff for 30 years. Giving this control to the resident may have to be done in a series of phases with appropriate training.

There is, of course, the danger that the above argument may be used to justify 'restrictive practices'. Practices carried out in a facility should match proper assessment of the individual's ability and needs. Thus, using a questionnaire such as 'The Hospital/ Hostels Practices Profile' in a facility designed according to a 'stepping stones' model, the number of practices described as 'restrictive' should decline, the more similar the section of the unit is to the community. Using the alternative model whereby support is gradually weaned off someone living in 'normal' accommodation, such practices can be a useful means of structuring this withdrawal of support appropriately. Further, getting the staff to fill out the questionnaire can be a useful exercise in making sure that the facility is monitoring its practices. It is also useful in seeing how different shifts adopt different practices.

As can be seen such issues as discussed above are very intricate and must be weighed up carefully. In many instances there are no 'right' or 'wrong' answers such as when 'to let go of somebody' who comes in and out of hospital many times, which could be avoided by careful follow-up which he/she decides to refuse.

LINKS WITH THE COMMUNITY

Apart from locating an appropriate building within the community, it is essential to foster links with local people to avoid 'attitudinal' isolation. It may even be useful to carry out some of the groundwork before the establishment is open. Even when it is running it might be appropriate to investigate attitudes to the unit and compare them with those to 'ordinary' community facilities. A survey can be carried out investigating attitudes to a number of facilities so as not to alarm the residents living nearby nor 'pick out' the main unit under study. Thus, for example, from a survey carried out on residents living near our own hostel and day-centre, Middlewood House, we learnt that many people were unaware as to what it was. Attitudes to it were basically positive and similar to a community centre nearby: despite sixteen articles in the local press in about as many months about it, most people's information about the facility came from small posters advertising jumble sales. An interesting finding was that despite overall positive attitudes, mothers of children under eleven were unsure about the place, hence the brownies using the community room for the meetings to try to break down this attitude. In trying to break down barriers between these community facilities and the community, a number of steps may be taken bearing in mind that the facility is the residents' home.

(1) Outsiders (such as families and friends) should be encouraged to come into the hostel. Volunteers may be used to befriend residents who are likely to remain there (at least in the first instance) especially if they would have difficulty getting to the community for whatever reason. The use of rooms by local groups can further help to break down barriers and help dispel the mistaken impression that the residents or day attenders are 'dangerous'. Activities like jumble sales can also help reduce any isolation.

(2) Further residents must be *encouraged* to go out into the community and use community facilities. I write '*encouraged*' because sometimes they are *forced*. This means that for hostels they should go out to get their medication rather than nursing staff come in to give it to them, thus turning the place into a mini-hospital. Similarly, residents should be encouraged to go to

the doctor for appointments and prescriptions rather than have the doctor visit them. For both these groups of professionals a guiding rule is what would happen in the community in someone's own home. Thus, if one could not get to the doctor because one was too incapacitated then one would expect him or her to call and not otherwise. In the first stages of a resident's stay one would arrange for a member of staff to go with them (or even another resident) rather than have the doctor call in. Likewise, residents should be encouraged to go out to the hairdressers and similar people rather than have them visit.

To encourage the interchange between the community and the unit it is important that the staff are aware and monitor what community facilities there are around them. Day-centres in particular should be wary of duplicating what is available outside. Thus, if there is a badminton group outside, then day attenders should be encouraged to use it rather than set one up in the day-centre. However, in some cases it may be appropriate to have a little duplication. In such cases one is aiming at *overlap* rather than *direct duplication*. Thus, when trying to help people with difficulties in reading and writing it may be appropriate to set up a special class to assist the clients with their confidence until they feel able to attend the ordinary lessons. Thus, the day-centre should be working in tandem with adult education facilities, community, and sports centres, to provide an overlap service to help integrate its clients into their facilities.

CO-OPERATION BETWEEN THE SERVICES

One of the underlying assumptions of 'community care' is that there is a will for agencies involved to co-operate, so as to transfer the emphasis of psychiatric care into the community. At the planning and management level health authorities should co-operate to transfer resources to local authorities. At present there does not appear to be much evidence that this is happening. Without co-operation at the planning level one gets duplication of services (for example, similar day-centres and day hospitals established in the same locality). Similarly, lack of services may result in inappropriate planning. Care Planning Teams are often merely reduced to bargaining shops with staff from both sides 'bartering' and making bids for joint financing money to prop up services they should be providing anyway.

At the service level hospital staff should help train individuals to return to the community. Unfortunately, this implies that Health Service staff may lose their jobs or at the very least their status. Health Service staff are worried that as the hospital runs down they might be made redundant. Further, they fear that if community staff are able to cope with the people formerly 'needing' hospitals then their nursing skills become devalued. One of their commonest complaints, however, is that staff in the community 'cream' off the easiest cases whilst leaving the hardest one behind and claim the credit for quick successes.

Community staff, however, may also fear 'community care' for they become worried that the Health Service will 'dump' their problem residents or what they might regard as 'long-stay no-hopers' on them and will not be prepared to take them back. They may also be concerned that Health Service staff could play 'Big Brother' on them and turn their hostels or day-centres into annexes of the hospital.

This lack of co-operation leads to:

(1) 'Borderline candidates' get shuttled between the two services (for example, people with severe behaviour problems).
(2) Health Service staff find difficulty in discharging people into the community and so their rehabilitation and pre- discharge units become blocked.
(3) Community Services facilities have low occupancy and 'turnover' rates since they do not take all the people they could.
(4) Health Service staff becoming unwilling to re-admit or give support to community staff and so leading to them and the people they are trying to help suffering.
(5) Community Service staff become unwilling to take people in a preventative role because they fear they may become 'stuck' with them.

There are a number of strategies which might avoid such difficulties and encourage co-operation.

(1) 'Catchment areas' should be sorted out such that staff from both services know who is responsible for whom. In our own

system, for example, one Social Services hostel has been set up in our catchment area which services another psychiatric hospital as well, whilst another hostel which also services both of us is in *that* hospital's catchment area. Such an arrangement could become fraught with difficulties. Should someone discharged from our hospital going into the second hostel turn to that other hospital in times of difficulties? Clearly, 'care in the community' should imply continuity of care and so agreements should be made to waive ordinary boundaries in such cases.

(2) Administration differences should be sorted out so that staff from both units should be aware of them and they should be minimized by allowing staff as much autonomy as possible. Hence, admission decisions should be left at unit level rather than at a placement section or at headquarters of a Social Services Department.

(3) Joint policies could be worked out between the units to allow easy 'flow through' where appropriate and to be criteria based so that one knows what is required.

(4) Co-operation between services is enhanced if both speak the same language – for example, using similar assessment forms, similar admission and discharge procedures.

(5) Even with such systems of co-operation it is helpful to have at least one member of staff who works at both places. This also helps prevent 'dumping' and 'creaming'. Such staff as well as easing the flow of information (the lack of which flaws many systems) can act as 'referee' in times of difficulty. My own post as a joint financed clinical psychologist, for example, was useful in the establishment of our joint system in preventing such difficulties becoming too serious.

(6) Visits to each other's units can be useful and can extend to an interchange scheme such as in our own system where residential social workers spend three weeks working at the hospital in return for nursing staff being placed at the hostel. It must be noted that nursing staff do not work at the hostel as traditional nurses but use it as an opportunity to extend their skills in working in a non-medical setting. Similarly the social workers get to learn the hospital system and what led to the residents coming to them. It is also useful to visit other systems as a joint team to learn how others

co-operate as well. Such trips often have a social element and are useful in building up face-to-face contacts. Allied to this last point it is useful for any presentations or symposia to be given jointly to help cement the system closer together.

(7) Joint training of staff with plenty of emphasis on practical interactive exercises can also be extremely useful. In our own system we run a week's course in (re)habilitation which is open to staff from our health, social, and voluntary units. Giving a training manual out to staff beforehand and short introductory 'talks' before each session leaves plenty of time for these co-operative tasks. Other opportunities for sharing of ideas (for example, representation on each other's planning committees) can encourage real 'on the ground' co-operation.

(8) It is crucial in establishing a co-operative system to set up a framework for overall evaluation. All too often if any review is carried out it is only devoted to part of the system. Thus, the Health Service side will have its own statistics which will be independent of those from the Social and Voluntary Services. Such a myopic approach ignores the interactive nature of 'community care'. The hospital that displays impressive discharge rates may be guilty of putting an inappropriate burden on the community. The Social Services rehabilitation hostel boasting a high throughput rate may have a high proportion of its clients being re-admitted back to the hospital. A joint evaluative system helps identify how much the service is really complimentary. For example, does the hostel and rehabilitation ward take the same people and if so does one need both or do you need to revise their functioning? Such an approach also helps identify those people who fall in between the services and what gaps there are in your system.

(9) Finally, joint social events can be a most useful means of staff from different units getting to know each other in a relatively non-threatening manner. This can be by parties or by monthly trips to a different restaurant by members of the various Health, Social, and Voluntary Service units as we do. It does not matter if everybody comes from the different units as long as there are at least some people from each section at this 'dining club'. Such informal gatherings can lead to any difficulties, aggravation, or rumour being cleared up in a non-threatening manner.

CONCLUSION

Unfortunately, there seems to be an idea prevalent that merely 'pointing people in the right direction should be sufficient to get an appropriate system of 'community care'. I have attempted to show in this chapter that it must be planned and not left to chance. Indeed, if one leaves it to develop in an haphazard fashion there is the danger that whenever practical difficulties are encountered, the will to co-operate may become subordinate to the feeling that one has been 'put upon', since it is a strain to set up a whole system which must be geared to an all-day and every-day service.

Although I have just touched upon many issues in this relatively brief discussion, I hope I have given some food for thought. 'Care in the Community' must be planned properly and I have tried to give some suggestions from my own experience of our own system and that of others. Although we were designated a National Demonstration Service in Rehabilitation because of the reasonably close co-operation between our services, we have made many mistakes and have a long way to go to achieve the system we would like. A will to co-operate is an essential precursor. Next is a framework for planning and sorting out any difficulties involving planners/managers and 'direct-care staff'. Thirdly, it is crucial that members of the various disciplines and agencies are more involved in the task at hand than their own professional interests. Finally, all these are subordinate to the needs and wishes of those we serve; the focus of 'Care in the Community'. Whilst much of the interest directed at the House of Commons Select Committee on Social Services Report (1985) has focused on the lack of community facilities, it is essential that they are appropriate. The danger is that more buildings and staff will be provided inappropriately, thereby bringing 'institutionalization' from the old Victorian hospitals along with the patients discharged into the community, thus turning 'Care in the Community' into 'Institutionalization in the Community'.

REFERENCES

Cochrane, R. (1983) *The Social Creation of Mental Illness*, London: Longman.

Department of Health and Social Security (1975) *Better Services for the Mentally Ill*, London: HMSO.

House of Commons (1985) *Second Report from the Social Services Committee: Community Care*, London: HMSO.

West Midlands Regional Health Authority Rehabilitation Survey Team (1979) *First Annual Survey of Rehabilitation Facilities in Hospitals for the Mentally Ill and Mentally Handicapped*, Birmingham: WMRHA.

Working Party of the Social Services Liaison Group (1978) *Report – Residential Care: Staffing and Training*, Birmingham: British Association of Social Workers

Chapter Seven

IMPLICATIONS FOR STAFF

How far can retraining go?

FRANCES BROWN

INTRODUCTION

Why do we train staff in human services? One reason, perhaps, is to make those staff feel better about the job they are doing. Another reason is that it may help those staff who are involved in offering the training to feel better. Everyone can feel they are involved in supporting each other, improving one another's learning, and so on. It is often easy in this way to pay lip- service to training and continue the lack of clarity about what we are trying to achieve by training.

Another reason why we train staff and which is clearly recognized by many, but not all, services, is to make those who receive the service from those staff feel better. If this is the prime reason it is clearer to see the role of training in the overall aim of services to best meet the needs of their consumers and to promote the best quality of life for them. One way to think of this is that if staff who receive training feel better about their job, more confident about what they are doing, they will offer a better quality of service than staff who feel depressed, devalued, and so on. I am also supposing that we see training as an integral part of a service and not as something quite separate with little relevance to implementation. At this point, I must stress that by training I am referring to any activity which comes under the heading of in-service training, post-basic training, staff development, induction training, re-training, use of external training consultants, and so on. Thus, in exploring the question 'How far can training/retraining go?', we need to assume that training includes all of these; and also that the implications of training for

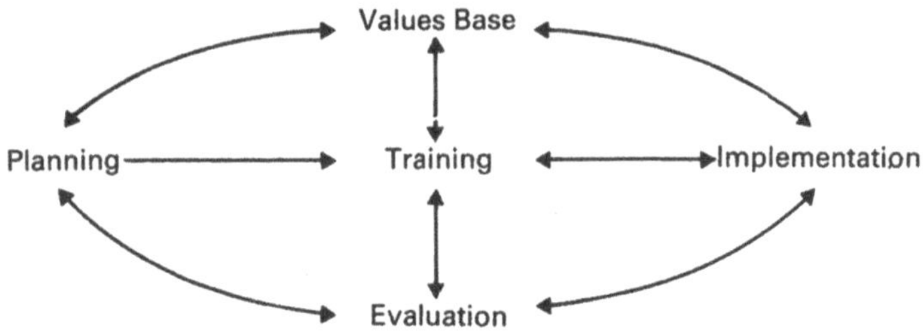

Figure 7.1 A context for staff training in human services

staff are about ensuring them a future in a high-quality service for consumers.

I must also stress that I assume all levels of staff require regular ongoing opportunities to re-evaluate and develop their knowledge, attitudes, skills, and their awareness of new ideas and new resources, and so on. I also assume that this applies irrespective of the service in which staff work – i.e. new and developing or traditional and contracting services, whether in health, education, social services settings, or voluntary organizations.

Training can, therefore, play a major role in the creation of a high-quality service with and for the consumers of that service *if* it is in touch with the different elements that constitute that service. Thus, the context of training and the interaction of these different elements is crucial.

This is a constantly evolving and developing picture with all these different aspects mutually influencing each other.

There are some clear implications arising from this view of a service context. First, there needs to be a clearly communicated statement of the service's *values base.* This must be freely available to all, consumers and service providers. This straight information-sharing is often a good starting-point in training.

Second, those *planning* the service must develop a strategy which clearly shows the process by which the values base will interact with the identified need and thus create the service framework. There are some key elements in the planning which training can help to highlight and about which it can share ideas and information. These include issues about the comprehensiveness of the strategy – is it intended to provide a service for everyone, irrespective of their degree of handicap? Also, is the service going to be provided for everyone within their locality – with no-one being sent away to receive services elsewhere? In addition, it needs to be clear whether the service is going to offer appropriate support, when needed, for all aspects of life for a person with a mental handicap. Other important elements addressed in planning should be the decisions about the roles of the various key personnel in offering the service, developing a balance between the contracting and the developing services, ensuring a continuity of service to the consumers, and communicating what the intended time-scale will be. Such a strategy clearly highlights the interactive role of training in this process. A good example of a strategy for services which also emphasizes the role of training is the 'Model District Service' (North Western Regional Health Authority 1983).

Third, *implementation* is where the values base and the planning process are put into direct action. If the skills necessary to implement the service are lacking at this point then all of the work of the two previous elements will count for nothing. It is, therefore, crucial that training has been provided which ensures a blend between the development of the appropriate values and skills in a complementary manner. The sorts of skills required are many and will vary from service to service. However, some will be common to all services – for example, management skills, problem-solving, imparting skills to others, communication and relationship skills, and so on.

Finally, *evaluation* of a service ensures that the impact of the service on its consumers is monitored and evaluated. Many organizations are exploring methods of achieving this. One possible way of doing this is through 'Quality Action Groups' (Independent Development Council 1986).

It is, therefore, clear that good-quality in-service training is an important thread running through these aspects of services and can ensure that they are kept in balance, by bringing the relevant people together to share their ideas, knowledge, and so on, and keep everyone aware of their respective roles.

While looking at the context for training it is worth looking at one particular area where an additional detail comes into play.

This is the personnel and manpower planning implications of the move from institutional to local ordinary services. Nationally, there seems to have been considerable effort put into the design of new services but little work done on how this interacts with the subsequent mass movement of, and changes for, staff.

The relationship between this and training is important for several reasons. In terms of planning how much training is required, manpower planning needs to make available as much information as possible on how many staff there are now in services, how many will be needed in the future developing services, and how many staff will require training, how much, and of what nature. This then requires an examination of the potential redeployment of staff geographically – perhaps from rural areas where many of the traditional services have been based to urban centres of population and the resulting impact on those staff. It also involves thought being given to the range of new jobs which may be created, for example employment/job finders, and how specific training can be geared to them. There may also be a debate about costs of redeploying and retraining versus redundancy costs. This is not just a financial question; it is also about the possible costs of losing experienced (albeit in traditional settings) staff.

Leading on from this, it then becomes apparent that staff in contracting services need to know their future role in maintaining a good quality of life for consumers of their service if 'ghetto services' are not to be created. It is possible that already the patterns for these 'ghetto services' are being set – namely, that new, younger staff who have had more exposure to the philosophies and values inherent in the new services are leaving the traditional settings. Those staff remaining may be 'digging in' either because they believe that hospital run-downs 'will never happen' – or because they will be entitled to redundancy/retirement when it does inevitably happen. If, as is also happening in some areas, this is coupled with receiving districts only resettling the more able people requiring less staff support, then the implications for those remaining are obvious. In this scenario it would seem that there would be a limited amount which training could do to resolve the situation for either service consumers or service providers if it becomes too advanced.

However, training does have a role to play in drawing attention to these possibilities. A final reason, which I will not discuss in detail, but is still another very significant reason for addressing manpower implications, is that of influencing future qualification-training. There needs to be a clear grasp of what kind of basic training staff in the new services will need – for example, social work or nurse training or something new and different? Is this going to be provided by the training available? - for example, the new Qualifying Diploma in Social Work (Central Council for Education and Training in Social Work 1986) or the new-style nursing training envisaged in Project 2000 (UKCC 1986). How many trained staff will be needed in the new services and can the training courses presently in existence provide sufficient numbers? Many of the lessons learned from in- service training may begin to point to some possible answers.

A major reason for ensuring that the personnel and manpower planning context is addressed is that staff will only take part in, learn, and benefit from training if they are assured on certain points. They must be given clear, concise, and increasingly detailed information about what the new services are going to look like. They need to know if jobs within these new services will be open to them – and if they are, how many jobs there will be, where they will be located and when they will become available. Staff need to be given information on what skills and abilities will be expected of those working in new services. They also need to know that they will have protected conditions of service if they do move jobs. Lastly, they need assurances that appropriate supports will exist for staff while they are changing jobs. Recently, more attention has been given to the needs of people with a mental handicap during their move from traditional settings to new, community-based settings with a growing awareness of the impact it has, the transitional shock, and so on. It should be an obvious step to recognize that staff will suffer from similar transitional problems and devise appropriate supports.

Therefore, a massive task exists for personnel staff in health, social services, and education authorities to work together in sharing information and to work in parallel with training and service developers. If this does not happen then no amount of training will prevent a large number of staff becoming depressed and demoralized and the corresponding waste of resources that this represents.

CONTENT OF TRAINING

The training provided, therefore, must also build on and recognize the *existing* skills, knowledge, and abilities which staff already have and which they could bring to new services. These may have been acquired in different ways, for example:

- basic qualification training;
- their experiences as a service provider;
- by being a member of a local community;
- by having special interests in particular areas – for example, leisure interests;
- through any special relationships developed with an individual consumer.

Some of these may be more relevant than others to the needs of people with a mental handicap requiring support in developing a new life in their local community. Access to skilled and sensitive training can help individual members of staff feel confident about building on their existing appropriate skills and learning about and developing the new ones they do not yet have.

This way of thinking about the individual training needs of staff should sound familiar to those working with people with a mental handicap and who are using strengths/needs lists, goal plans, individual programme plans, and so on. These ideas can be equally well applied to people who are service providers and can then provide guidelines about how to structure training. The In-Service Training staff at Calderstones Hospital in Lancashire have used this format in their document 'Staff Training in Resettlement' (Calderstones 1987).

It can be argued, therefore, that the content of training must contain a blend of the following three areas. The first is straight information sharing – staff must have opportunities to know how the new services will look and their content. They must be clear about how quality will be maintained in the contracting services. In addition, there must be access to information about new ideas and approaches which are being developed and which they will be expected to help implement. This can be offered in regular briefing sessions which are open to all levels and categories of staff and must be well advertised.

Second, the area of values and attitudes must be looked at. Staff need time, space, and support to explore their own and the service's values and then to work out any possible conflicts. This can be offered in the form of workshops, preferably over two or three days, introducing the Principle of Normalization, which gives people the opportunity to be clear about what the Principle actually is and not to assume that it means 'making people normal' – which is a common misunderstanding where there has been no workshop available.

Last, but most definitely not least, training must be available which ensures and enhances the development of the necessary skills. These may include areas such as:

- listening;
- communication;
- management of new developing services;
- management of traditional, contracting services;
- teaching skills to people with mental handicaps – for example, social skills, practical skills, relationship skills (including sexuality);
- the role of staff in supporting self-advocacy;
- supporting individuals in informed choice;
- working with people with challenging behaviour;
- use of ordinary local or generic resources.

These 'skill' workshops can take many forms. Some may be in-house – with staff from one particular setting all taking part. Another way is to send one or two staff to external courses and on their return to communicate with their colleagues about what they have learned. The learning may be generalized and open to many staff from different services or they may be specific to one individual consumer or a small group of people and be made available to the key worker or workers.

SOME COMPONENTS FOR A SUCCESSFUL TRAINING STRATEGY

If training is going to be significant in improving services for both consumers and providers then it has to take part, not only within the context described above, but it must also be part of a coherent training strategy. This strategy must have several crucial components. First, there has to be commitment across all services and at all levels that training is important. This leads to clarity about the need to provide resources for training – not just about the obvious financial costs of training but also the hidden costs in releasing staff without detriment to the service consumers.

Another important component is the existence of local joint training groups, preferably with some 'clout' – for example, by being formal subgroups of Joint Care Planning teams. These groups work best when they have a varied membership which includes representatives from all the agencies in the area responsible for services for people with mental handicap. Within this there should be a blend of service providers, managers, and trainers. Increasingly, the joint training groups which are working well are ensuring that consumers, direct and/or secondary, are also full and valued members, as well as contributing to, and taking part in, training events. Joint training groups can avoid duplication by communicating about their various in-house resources. They can then work together to share these resources – namely, people, skills, budgets, venues, and so on. This then leads to the best and most efficient use of all of these resources in a locality.

The next component is an awareness of the need to balance the different methods of training. This means deciding on the relative benefits of sending one or two staff away on expensive external courses for some aspects of service developments with closing down a whole site and ensuring all staff participate in an 'on-site' workshop – and the various styles of training intervention in between. Another component is ensuring that induction training is *always* followed by on-going, in- service training and is not a one-off event which whets appetites and then leaves people with raised expectations which eventually turn to disappointment or cynicism.

A successful training strategy also ensures that best use is made of external training supports. This could be anything from one-day events to longer courses offered by organizations such as the Central Council for Education and Training in Social Work (CCETSW), the English National Board (ENB), the British Institute for Mental Handicap (BIMH), Regional Training Teams (Training Team for Mental Handicap Services 1986). It also includes decisions about packages for training such as those available from the Open University or ESCATA, and so on. Finally, a good training strategy ensures that there is a commitment for all staff to have the time and space to explore new ideas and approaches, in a safe and supported way.

If training does take place within the appropriate context and strategy it then implicitly also plays an important role in promoting contact between various groups of people. These include:

- consumers and staff;
- staff from different agencies;
- staff from all levels of a service;
- staff from contracting services and those in developing services;
- staff and consumers from different areas;
- basic training courses and in-service training.

As well as promoting better understanding and communication, all of these contacts can ensure the continuing interplay among, and influencing of, the major elements of a service.

CONCLUSION

In conclusion, any attempt to address the original question of 'How far can training/retraining go?' means giving a qualified answer. It can only contribute to a positive future for staff if certain conditions exist. First, there has to be a clear, well- communicated strategy for service planning, development, and implementation. This needs to be accompanied by a coherent personnel and manpower planning strategy. Within these there also needs to be a specific training strategy which is joint with all agencies and clearly spelt out for all staff. Also, the training provided must provide a blend of information sharing, values- based training, and a range of skill development training; all of which are ongoing and developing with the service. There must also be a recognition of the existing skills which staff have – especially in the contracting services. Following on from this point it is important that training provides a forum for staff from both traditional contracting and new, developing services. They can then be learning and training together and from each other.

Finally, but probably most importantly, training can go a long way to improve the situation for staff *if* it is improving the service for consumers. The best way of achieving this, and determining that this continues, is to ensure that consumers, both direct and secondary, are fully participating, involved, and consulted partners.

REFERENCES

Calderstones (1987) 'Staff Training in Resettlement'.
Central Council for Education and Training in Social Work (1986) 'Three years and different routes', Paper 20.6.
Independent Development Council (1986) 'Pursuing Quality', London: IDC (126 Albert Street, NW1 7NF).
North Western Regional Health Authority (1982) 'A Model District Service'.
Training Team for Mental Handicap Services – North Western Regional Health Authority (1986) 'Report on Staff Development and Training Initiatives'.
United Kingdom Central Council (1986) 'Project 2000 – A New Preparation for Practice'.

Chapter Eight

SIMILARITIES AND DIFFERENCES BETWEEN CLIENT GROUPS

Values and myths

IAN MACDONALD

This chapter draws on two models. First, a model for understanding change process (Macdonald 1989, forthcoming) and second, a model for understanding values and mythologies (Macdonald and Stewart 1989, forthcoming). This latter model, based on work by K. Stewart in Australia, allows for an examination of the assumptions which form the basis of past and current practice with regard to service provision.

The majority of services for client groups are and always have been provided 'in the community'. Most people, whether they are regarded as mentally ill, handicapped, or simply old do not end up living in large institutions. This has always been a back-stop or an asylum when families, friends, or services can no longer provide for people in the community. However, significant numbers of people have spent much, if not all, of their lives separated from 'normal' life. Current stated policy (DHSS 1982) at all levels is for the reduction of 'institutional' services and the development of community-based services (King's Fund 1980). There is an articulated belief that this move will be beneficial to client groups. In the field of mental handicap the principles of 'normalization' (Wolfensberger 1972) have influenced this process and particularly emphasized the rights of people with a mental handicap.

Such a policy does not effectively discriminate between client groups. The general principles are based on universal rights and similarities, not differences. The demand for services that are based on individual need is also common for all groups. The contrast is made between an individually designed programme of care being delivered to a person (and family) in a normal house and that of a standard, routine system being delivered to an anonymous person who is indistinguishable from all the others in a large institution.

It has been argued elsewhere that changes in provision for such groups have been motivated more by a general concern for humane conditions and administrative convenience, rather than a real understanding of the particular needs of such people (Macdonald 1989, forthcoming). How might we examine whether this time we are really improving the lives of people in such groups? One feature in the provision of care for such groups is that many members of such groups are not able, used, or allowed to express their own views with sufficient clarity. It is not simply a question of asking them what they would like. Applying techniques of market research in this field is hardly straightforward. Although much work has been done in the field of self-advocacy and parental/family participation, this does not in itself solve the problem as a significant proportion of such groups still rely on others to speak on their behalf. Indeed, if they could express themselves clearly most would not need the service. Second, discussions of service provision and needs are not simple, rational occasions. It is a feature of such services that they appropriately raise a great deal of emotion and strong views. Caring for such groups still contains a vocational element. Phrases such as 'improved quality of life' are not easy to translate into universally accepted criteria. Contradictory arguments are presented concerning the same circumstances. The fact that a person has been in a hospital for 30 years leads to an assumption that either it would be cruel to take them out, away from a familiar life and surroundings or it is about time they were let out and given at least some chance to lead a better life. After all, the fact that someone has served a 25-year sentence is no justification for keeping that person in prison even longer.

The field is heavily influenced by beliefs, values, opinions and attitudes, and it is naïve to assume that a rational planning process alone will convince people to change. Given the context of a drive for care in the community, this chapter seeks to examine the processes which link behaviour and values. If changes in service provision are to occur, then people providing services and receiving them are required to change their behaviour. From previous work by the author (1989, forthcoming) and Macdonald

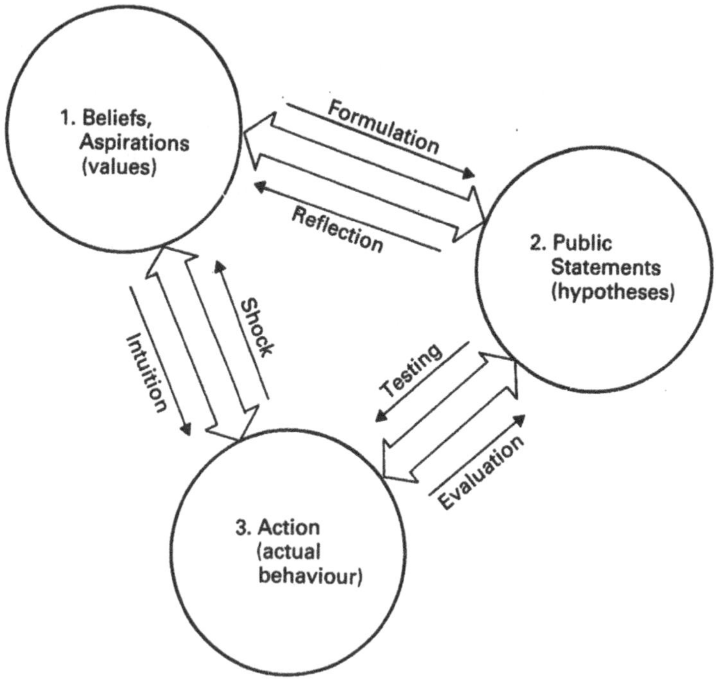

Figure 8.1 A model for understanding change process

and Stewart (1989, forthcoming) and psychological theory in general, it is proposed that rational argument alone does not guarantee change. People are not convinced solely by facts and figures; it depends whether they think or want to think that such facts and figures represent the 'truth' and whether they believe and trust the person presenting the facts and figures. At the other extreme, however, people may be convinced solely by the emotional 'arguments', by irrational belief systems which are congruent with their own need.

One model for examining this change process is set out in Figure 8.1 (Macdonald 1989, forthcoming). In this model *beliefs* are largely implicit, they give a general direction to behaviour. They determine our orientation to the world. However, they may be articulated into a set of clear *statements* or *hypotheses* which in turn can be tested in *action*. The interactions between these elements determine the rate and amount of change in the system as a whole. I may have a belief, for example, that people from Scotland are mean. I may turn that into a specific hypothesis that a particular Scotsman will avoid paying for a round of drinks when it is his turn. I then have to test this in action. If he does pay, without hesitation, I must modify my belief in some way. Here the maintenance of the original belief produces cognitive dissonance which is difficult to maintain. I may of course turn this belief into an untestable prejudice, to maintain my original belief in the face of 'evidence'. Thus, for example, he is not really a Scot (his mother was part English), or he guessed I was testing him, or the ultimate escape: 'he is the exception which proves the rule'.

This model is put forward in order to test some of the current thinking in service delivery. What are the beliefs that underpin the service? i.e. 'philosophies', 'rights', and so on. How are they translated into testable hypotheses and what are these hypotheses? Finally, are they modified in the light of actual behaviour – i.e by evaluation? The model is also presented to demonstrate the implication of avoiding one of these elements. To ignore *beliefs* and values produces an amoral approach, apparently based on a rational 'scientific' model but actually devoid of essential human characteristics of motivation and intention. To ignore *action* is to produce a set of theories and hypotheses which are never adequately tested. It leads to the pejorative meaning of 'academic' and 'theory' and the split of practice from thought.

To ignore *hypotheses*, i.e. to move directly from belief to action, is exemplified by strong charismatic leaders with unquestioning followers or doers. Parts of the service are influenced by this approach, full of emotion and energy, but they wither when the charismatic leader leaves since the formulation or link between belief and action has not been expressed in a form which can be tested, altered, or even carried out by someone else.

The importance of formulation is to make the process independent of specific individuals; as such it can be a direct threat to personal power. Essentially, formulation takes away the magic; demystifies the process. However, we cannot formulate everything. Life is not a scientific experiment and providing services to client groups is not simply a means of testing hypotheses. Consequently, there are many different opinions concerning how best to meet the needs of clients. It is not possible to test all of these systematically and broad generalizations and assumptions may become guiding principles. Concepts such as 'family living', 'group homes', 'village communities', 'community living', are subsets of more general movements such as 'normalization' or 'institutional care', but not necessarily clearly defined.

It now seems to be accepted that in order to change behaviour it is necessary to change attitudes. However, there is a set of concepts which are not easily distinguished. These are 'attitudes', 'values', 'beliefs', and 'philosophies'. Policies are often preceded by 'philosophies of care' which contain statements of values and rights. They sometimes take the form of a small bill of rights or constitution: 'we hold these truths to be self-evident'. These are necessary to ensure that the service givers share the same views as to the overall purpose of their action. Such documents often refer to the treatment of people with dignity, equal value, including rights of access to community facilities (King's Fund 1980).

From work in Australian industry, Stewart and the present author propose a model which attempts to clarify some of the confusions which arise from associating behaviour directly with value statements. The model is discussed in more detail elsewhere (Macdonald and Stewart 1989, forthcoming) but essentially argues that values and behaviour are not linked in a fixed way. Indeed, if behaviour becomes irrevocably associated with a value, the society or culture becomes rigid and gives rise to repressive ideologies. The emergence of such a rigid ideology of care for client groups leads to an unquestioning approach in which critics are associated with negative values.

The model argues that for any society to continue to exist there is a basic set of values which guide behaviour. Behaviour which is perceived to demonstrate these values is accorded worth, that is, it is seen to be acceptable behaviour, and behaviour which is accorded negative worth and is perceived to demonstrate the negative value is unacceptable. The basic set of values in their abstract form, which as far as we can determine are cross-cultural, are as follows: love, trust, courage, dignity, fairness, and honesty.[1] They are not in any order of priority. We argue that all societies or organized groups can only continue to exist and develop by assigning worth to those members who demonstrate behaviour in accordance with the basic value set. Conversely, societies try to control and discourage behaviour which demonstrates their opposites, i.e. behaviour which is unloving, mistrusting, cowardly, undignifying, unfair, and dishonest. 'Societies' may be nations, businesses, services, or any organized group.

The problem arises when determining which behaviour demonstrates positive or negative values. At any one time a group may agree implicitly or explicitly which behaviour demonstrates the positive or negative of the values. We argue that this association is a mythology. It is not possible to determine absolutely the real intention of an individual (particularly if it is accepted that we have unconscious motives). What we do in general terms is to ascribe intentions to a behaviour, which can be more rigorously tested (if necessary) in an individual case. Let us take an example from the field of mental handicap. In the process of preparing an individual plan, should the person with a mental handicap be present? There is a strong argument that decisions about such clients in the past have been made without their knowledge or involvement. To use the value set, such behaviour has been seen as unloving, unfair, untrusting, and undignifying towards the person with a mental handicap. Therefore there is an argument that they should be included. However, another mythology might argue that to *include* the person is undignifying (since they can be overwhelmed by the discussion), that it is dishonest since it pretends that the person is of equal ability, and cowardly since the carers do not have the courage to make up their own minds. The point of this example is to demonstrate that it is not possible to prescribe that a particular set of behaviours will guarantee agreement concerning the demonstration of positive values.

It is not possible to avoid mythologies. We need to predict and assign personalities to likely behaviour. We must make certain assumptions or every behaviour would have to be examined in detail. We would enter every social relationship with complete uncertainty and these relationships would be cumbersome and time-consuming. The assignment of values to behaviour allows us to predict future relationships. If we see someone hit a client it provides information about that relationship and influences our relationship towards the participants. We assign a motive to the behaviour and determine the value that the person is demonstrating.

In general terms, systems, that is the formulated processes of relationships, all demonstrate values. Thus, for example, we have beliefs about individual programmes and plans, appraisal systems, selection systems, assessment systems, tests, and so on. We construct mythologies about them, that they are fair or unfair, treat us with dignity, and so on. The mythology allows us to categorize and assign value at high speed. It is unfair, for example, to allocate community places on the basis of an IQ test score; that it is unloving to break up friendships when people move to a different location; that to lock people up is cowardly and undignifying; to assume that people can be treated successfully by drugs is dishonest, and so on. In Australia some of these ideas have been tested in the field of the management of large mines (for example, iron ore, bauxite, coal). It was particularly interesting to examine the value set with regard to systems. There is an easy trap to fall into, i.e. that systems design is a technological process, particularly when using computers. It was demonstrated that far from systems being perceived as purely technological processes, they were the very embodiment of values. In one group, for example, the same systems of housing benefit, travelling expenses, and car allowance were seen as demonstrating (by some) the fairness and honesty of the company, and by others as a prime example of unfairness and lack of trust. The discussion concerning such boring, bureaucratic processes was highly emotive. Systems design (within the company: CRA)[2] is now receiving significant attention and it is done at a high level within the organization. The symbolic meaning of the system is recognized.

In the field of mental handicap the systems of individual planning also demonstrate the values of the organization. The impact of such systems, in terms of values and level of work, can easily be underestimated. The introduction of such systems is often seen as a process of teaching people how to fill in forms rather than raising the level of work, and ignores the current mythologies of the group (Macdonald et al. 1987).

However, we move to dangerous ground when we assume these mythologies to be facts – that is, when a particular behaviour or set of behaviours is automatically assumed to demonstrate a positive or negative value. In this way mythologies take on the force of a fundamental religion. If this process is applied to service provision, then 'normalization' could move from a set of mythologies and propositions to a belief system. People become priests and heretics. Unbelievers are shunned, outcasts from the now fundamental society which cannot tolerate dissent. This in turn splits (and eventually splinters) the society into sects which spend more time and energy on controlling its members and fighting enemies than developing ideas or getting on with its original purpose. Of course this is an analysis of the extreme case and not a necessary outcome.

Mythologies, as argued above, are necessary in order to increase predictability in relationships. In fact the existence of a coherent set of mythologies creates the culture of the society and allows for comfortable exchange between members. We need to have a reasonably predictable social environment in order to work and survive. If, however, we weld behaviour to values, then anyone who behaves (according to our mythology) in a way that demonstrates a negative value is a threat to society. An alternative perspective is to try and understand their mythology, or how they might interpret their behaviour in a positive light.

With regard to client groups, it may be that other people genuinely believe that a particular form of treatment or care, which we find abhorrent, is in their mythology actually demonstrating all the positive values. The alternative explanation of their behaviour is to assign motives of dishonesty, unfairness, lack of love, and so on to those individuals or groups. One common feature with regard to the different client groups is that their care, whether in 'hospitals', the community, Social Services, or voluntary establishments, increasingly involves multidisciplinary care. Now each profession could be regarded as a small society with its own culture or set of mythologies. Given the knowledge base and historical development of these professions, social work, physiotherapy, occupational therapy, speech therapy, psychiatry, educational and clinical psychology, music and art therapy, nursing, and so on, it is highly unlikely that they will all share the same culture or set of mythologies. However, they must all work together, hopefully with the overall purpose of benefiting the people they serve. If they have different mythologies then actual behaviours will lead to different interpretations with potential conflict between the professional 'societies' and confusion for the client.

The history of care is one in which professions have been in competition for a dominant mythology. Medicine, particularly psychiatry, in both mental illness and handicap, is no longer the unquestioned dominant profession. However, this can lead to a view that since the medical mythology has not prevailed, then anyone who still clings to it is untrustworthy, dishonest, unfair, and so on. Since, as has been argued above, these areas are at times highly emotional, the future of multidisciplinary work can be put in jeopardy. Professions and individuals can be ignored, their contributions literally devalued because they have a different mythology, and the client misses out again.

It is because we do not have many highly predictive theories, and consequently no single profession can guarantee outcomes of action, that there is a need for multidisciplinary involvement. Somewhere amongst this plethora of ideas from a wide collection of people including the clients, their families and representatives lies a helpful path towards an improved life with a more positive value.

LEADERSHIP

The leadership of such teams is a difficult process. I define leadership work as follows: 'The work of a leader is to articulate purpose and then to understand the dynamics of social process to enable constructive intervention.' By constructive intervention I mean that the leader should be able to stimulate or inspire behaviour which leads to the achievement of the group's purpose. This cannot be done without an understanding of the group dynamics. Applying the values model, a leader should therefore have the ability to perceive and understand the underlying mythologies of the groups concerned: that is, to appreciate the possibility that genuine differences may occur and that this does *not* mean that the profession or individuals concerned have a different set of values. It is critical for the leadership to determine between competing mythologies, i.e. genuine disagreement and when an individual really is being dishonest, one can easily obscure the other.

In this process the leader must demonstrate two abilities: first, the ability to create an overarching mythology, and second, consistently to behave in ways which are congruent with it. If the leader (individual or group, for example profession) demonstrates unloving or untrustworthy behaviour according to the overarching mythology, then the whole approach is discredited.

Currently, the need to go back to basics, to formulate 'philosophies' with policy statements (as mentioned above) is the attempt to create an overarching set of mythologies or culture which is acceptable to all and has direct benefit to the recipient of the service. The overarching current philosophy or culture in the field of mental handicap is that of 'normalization' with its PASS (Programme Analysis of Service Systems) training workshops.

A further requirement for leadership is the ability to create a culture which is so secure it can be questioned. This refers back to the first model presented. The culture must be open to formulation: that is, ideas need to be put in a testable form where outcomes or actions can be evaluated and the mythologies changed if necessary. If the culture is insecure or fundamentalist, then hypotheses and theories cannot be tested and developed. Vested interests develop which cannot sustain the possibility that village communities might have something to offer, or small group and independent living might have some drawbacks. In this way serious academic work is potentially threatening to society since it may require that the society alters its thinking and rejects some mythologies (Galileo was not exactly rewarded by the Church).

CONCLUSION

This chapter starts with the assumption that people delivering care to client groups are for the most part attempting to provide the best service possible. (Those who are shown not to be doing so have no part in the service). Partly because we have few predictive theories and partly because this area can be highly emotive there is a wide range of opinions as to the best way forward. This leads to disagreement among people which can be interpreted as people having 'different values or attitudes'. The chapter has attempted to argue that all of us actually share the same basic set of values. However, we differ in our association as to which behaviours express positive or negative value: i.e. we have different mythologies. If we assume these mythologies to be facts then we create fundamentalist cultures which will be in conflict with one another. This is the danger of turning models (for example, normalization) into quasi-religious ideologies with believers and heretics.

If multidisciplinary care is to be successful it requires a leadership which understands these various mythologies and the ability to turn at least some of these mythologies into testable formulations which can be properly evaluated. There is no simple way round this, i.e. by ignoring values or hypotheses or action. Finally, the last decade has seen a greater emphasis and concern to treat recipients of services with love, dignity, and honesty, to be fairer and more trusting, all of which at times requires courage. This improvement can be undermined if we do not treat colleagues, other professionals, and volunteers in the same way.

NOTES

1. Whether this is the best expression of the basic value set, i.e. whether there are 5, 6, or 7, is not the primary question and the exclusion of one or more is not the major issue. It is, rather, that there is a basis for assigning worth.
2. CRA Ltd., Collins Street, Melbourne 3001, Australia.

REFERENCES

DHSS (1982) *Care in the Community*, A Consultative Document for Moving Resources for Care in England, HMSO: London.

King's Fund (1980) 'An Ordinary Life', *Comprehensive locally based services for mentally handicapped people*. King's Fund Project Paper, no. 24, February, King's Fund Centre, London.

Macdonald, I. (1989, forthcoming) 'Services for whom?', in S. Baldwin (ed.) *Mental Handicap: Social Sciences Perspectives*, London: Croom Helm.

——and Stewart, K. (1989 forthcoming) *A Question of Values*, Mental Handicap Services Unit (MHSU) Publication, Brunel Institute of Organization and Social Studies (BIOSS), Brunel University.

Macdonald, I., Ovretveit, J., and Bein, T. (1987), *The Management of Change*, Epsom, Surrey: St Ebba's Mental Handicap Research Unit, St Ebba's Hospital.

Wolfensberger, W. (1972) *The Principle of Normalisation in Human Services*, Downsview, Toronto: National Institute on Mental Retardation.

Part Three

EXAMPLES OF GOOD PRACTICE

Chapter Nine

INDIVIDUAL SERVICES TO PEOPLE WITH PROFOUND MENTAL HANDICAPS AND CHALLENGING BEHAVIOUR

JAN HILL-TOUT

THE CHALLENGE

The clients

Malcolm is 23 years old. When he was 11 he was sent home from school with a note in his satchel saying 'please don't come back – we can't cope'. Malcolm stayed at home until he was 20, when his mother was finally persuaded that he could attend the Special Needs Department of the Adult Training Centre. Malcolm has spent a lot of his time at the ATC standing or walking around the room. He has no speech but a very loud scream of protest when he is unhappy. When approached by people, he may be affectionate but he may equally as well bite or scratch in a very unpredictable way. When he is at home Malcolm is excluded in a separate room when things are too bad and his mother is quite badly marked by him. His mother finds it hard to keep the home as she would like it because he is inclined to be destructive, doing things like pulling down curtains, tipping over the television, and throwing things.

Andrew is 26 years old. He lives at home with his parents and has attended the Special Needs Department of the ATC for several years. Until recently he spent much of his time walking about the room or standing and gazing out of the window. He also unpredictably went around the room throwing small and large objects, especially chairs. At home Andrew's parents' lives have been largely governed by him. They have been unable to keep their ornaments and furniture as they would like and have had polycarbonated glass fitted to the windows of their house. The most effective way they have found of dealing with Andrew's behaviour has been to take him out for a ride in the car, and this happens frequently when Andrew is at home in the evenings and weekends.

The strategy

The All Wales Strategy gives us a sound philosophical underpinning on which to base our work: an ordinary life in an integrated setting; the chance to be valued by others and to form genuine friendships; the opportunity to use community facilities and personal choices in how time is spent – things which are very difficult to achieve in an institutionalized setting but which most of us take for granted. To this end, therefore, we are gradually closing down segregated institutionalized services and replacing them with ordinary community activities. For the majority of mentally handicapped people this is a thoroughly achievable and valued aim. There is a well researched body of knowledge in the areas of ordinary housing, individual planning, and teaching new skills (NIMROD evaluations 1981–5). Given adequate funding and joint working, there is no reason why the ideas shouldn't become a reality for most mentally handicapped people, whatever their level of physical or mental handicap.

The challenge

But what of people like Andrew and Malcolm? Take Andrew to the supermarket and he will pull the tins off the shelves. Take Malcolm to the swimming pool and he might bite the swimmers. How are we going to give them the way of life to which they have a right in a genuine way. Not as spectators strapped into a wheelchair or held firmly by minders but as participants enjoying what they are doing and making their own contribution. This is the challenge with which the Rhondda Vanguard Service is grappling.

POSSIBLE ANSWERS

Relationships with others

The relationships that people like Andrew and Malcolm and hundreds of other people in hospitals and ATCs have with others are very peculiar. For the most part their interactions with others are blatantly coercive. People only approach them when they want them to do something – have a bath, eat a meal, get on a minibus. There is never much choice in the matter. Therapeutic interventions have tended to take the same form – do a puzzle, say a word, sit at a table for a length of time – well-intentioned guesses at what might be a useful skill to learn. To see the situation from another angle, because people like Malcolm and Andrew cannot communicate in the usual ways, they are forced into using fairly powerful coercive techniques to get what they want out of people – throwing objects, stripping, sitting on the floor, and so on. At no point does it occur to either person in the relationship to approach the other for company, or fun, or emotional warmth.

A new way of relating

What if people were given the space to develop these relationships? What if Andrew and Malcolm could have the chance to spend large chunks of time with another person in a situation where no-one was demanding anything. No goal-setting, no feeding programme, just unconditional time spent doing something enjoyable where escape is easy. For some of us this might be equated to having a drink with a friend, watching television with the family, doing a bit of window shopping, and so on.

Ideas into action

This approach has been tried with Andrew and Malcolm. Andrew was allowed a daily hour of individual time in his ATC setting. Space was allocated to him, along with a member of staff and some activities that it was thought he might enjoy. He was never forced to participate although he was given plenty of opportunities – he could come and go as he pleased. At first the staff member spent most of his time alone, but after 3 months Andrew was spending the full session seated at a table engaging in various activities and clearly enjoying himself. He started participating more in group activities during the rest of the day and his family found him easier to manage at home. Incidence of chair-throwing decreased and staff felt brave enough to take him swimming, to the pub, and on the train – with one-to-one and sometimes two-to-one support. Work with Malcolm has achieved similar results. He goes to a special sports session once a week and goes to a local cafe on the train. Malcolm and Andrew could have done all these things before but they would have been forced into it. There is a very long way to go of course but these are the small beginnings of a shift of focus in our work with these clients.

It is highly individualized and staff-intensive but more likely to lead to the sorts of constructive results in terms of our values that we would like to see. Basically it has allowed us to make realistic and achievable demands on each other because we now know each other – before we were just stabbing in the dark.

GETTING STARTED

Small is beautiful

The thought of giving chunks of individual time to large numbers of people can cause mental paralysis so it is a good idea to start small rather than not at all. Local negotiations can result in small reallocations of staff time and physical resources and this is all that is needed to get started. Small bits of high- quality work can be very contagious and can start people thinking in different ways. The work at Ely hospital in Cardiff has shown this (Hill-Tout 1985, 1988) and from small beginnings an individual service has been created to meet the needs of profoundly handicapped people and has been a very helpful model to the several community-based schemes now developing in South Wales.

Service implications

Within our own service in the Rhondda Vanguard area the service implications are massive but are being tackled in such a way as to make them manageable. Each incremental challenge to the service is based on a very concrete individual need, and so those involved in pursuing it are highly motivated to achieve results. Things that spring to mind are individual taxis for the very small number of people who may not be able to handle group transport arrangements, one-off allocations of finance to purchase special equipment for an individual rather than an institution, and plans for increasing and reallocating staff so that people do actually have the space in the day to spend time together and get to know each other. Experiences at Ely and the Rhondda have shown that a simplistic pragmatic approach like this can be very persuasive at various levels within a service.

THE FOLLOW ON

The beginning of an approach which has been described here does not tell us where to go next, and of course it cannot do so. When dealing with individuals, especially those who have developed unusual ways of relating to the world, we should be very wary of prescriptive approaches which usually stem from the services needs rather than the needs of the individual. Having said this, however, it would obviously be very foolish not to plan, if only to counteract the natural pull towards neat circumscribed answers.

A solution has to be found to the difficulties of issues like housing, leisure, and use of ordinary facilities. In our experience it will probably be necessary to pass through various grades of special services before a person can take part in the ordinary, and it is this gradation to which service planners should be sensitive, creating a service flexible enough to respond to changing need. It may be that some individuals actually need an interim safe environment between hospital and ordinary house, or that the ordinary house needs to be run in such a way as to limit choices at first. Perhaps day services should create quiet environments so that people are gradually exposed to the new experiences they have such trouble dealing with.

There is no easy answer but the bottom line is that the service should be responsive and work *with* the clients rather than *on* them. This is simply a perspective and will have different service implications according to the clients' needs. It seems to our team that the greatest demand this way of working makes on the service is not financial but in terms of team work at all levels and it is when this has broken down that matters have become most difficult.

SUMMARY

Work with two individuals living within the Rhondda has indicated that a good starting-point for working with people whose behaviour challenges us is to spend regular periods of unstructured non-coercive time together, simply to try and develop new ways of communicating. In doing this it is potentially easier to reach an understanding of needs, and ways in which service resources can be organized to meet those needs. From this starting-point exposure to new experiences and living situations can be achieved sensitively and incrementally, and service planners can use knowledge of individual need to create a service which is flexible enough to meet those needs in the long term.

REFERENCES

Hill-Tout, J. (1985) 'Daytime activity in hospital: two years on', *Journal of the British Institute of Mental Handicap* 13 (March): 30–2; (June): 78–9.

——(1988) 'Personal Services: an individual programme for a young mentally handicapped man', *Community Care* 697 (Feb.): 22–4.

Mental Handicap in Wales – Applied Research Unit (1981, 1982, 1983) 'Long term evaluation of services for mentally handicapped people in Cardiff: yearly reports'.

——(1985) 'Progress report'.

APPENDIX

There follows a verbatim transcription of an interview with Malcolm's mother. This interview describes life with Malcolm from her point of view, and in so doing highlights the complex nature of some of our clients' difficulties, and by implication the level of sophistication that service providers will need in their solutions.

TALKING TO MALCOLM'S MOTHER: MRS B.

QUESTION: When did you first notice there was something different about Malcolm?

Mrs B. Well, Malcolm was very slow in walking, slow in talking. At 2 years old he went into a kind of coma and started having fits, and he had brain damage after that. Nobody seemed to know what caused it. Nobody wanted to know. You know, I sent for the doctor. I had to send for him about three times the same day ... but he never said well we'll take him into hospital and find out what ... nothing. Once he went into that fit, he stopped talking completely.

QUESTION: What sort of advice and support did you receive?

Mrs B. None. I had to cope on my own with it. A social worker came when it was time for him to go to school, to see about letting Malcolm go to special school, and of course I had to let him go somewhere. He was about four. He didn't go to nursery ... nothing. He used to have terrible fits at that time. He was taking epinutin and phenobarbitones.

QUESTION: How did members of your family feel about the problems you were having with him?

Mrs B. Well, they helped all they could you know my father was terrible. My father worshipped him – he was the only boy. There was just my sister and myself, two girls, and my sister had two girls and he was the only boy. He was devastated. My parents have been wonderful. We used to go out a lot. Bill, my husband, wouldn't come with me anywhere you see. He wouldn't come anywhere with us, so it was always my father used to take Malcolm for a ride in the car. My father would be with me going for a walk, because people that didn't know about us always thought that my father was my husband. You know – my father never looked old, he was never grey or nothing and everybody thought he was my husband, because Bill wouldn't come with us.

QUESTION: What memories do you have of school days?

Mrs B. Not very happy ones I'm afraid. He went straight to the special school. He was with kids of his own age. I don't know what he did when he was there. They used to complain – he's still got the habit – when he gets tired he puts his hands down his trousers. He used to play with the pin, he did, on his nappy. Of course they complained about that so I had to have special suits made – cat suits. He had to wear cat suits to school. He came home one day – my father went berserk. He came home one day – he used to have a lot of petitmals as well, and he always used to fall backwards. Well, he came home one day and, I'm not exaggerating, he had a lump on the back of his head like that cup. One of the teachers only lived around the corner so I went down. They hadn't noticed it. So I said come on, you know, I'm not saying they could help it because I know he used to fall but to send him home and not say a word about it. I didn't like him going there at all, but where could he go?

QUESTION: Did they used to restrain him at school?

Mrs B. Like I said, an ordinary dining chair. They used to put him to sit – turn him around so his legs were through the back of the chair. So he couldn't get out – he couldn't get up and walk, because the back of the chair would be facing him. There was no way he could get from there. When he came home from school with his satchel – he used to take two nappies in a satchel – I said oh I said there's a letter in here and it said not to send him back after half-term because they couldn't cope with him. So I phoned and I said can you tell me why. Now at that time I know he was terrible, I know, but they reckon it took five of them to change his nappy. Well I said I've got to do it on my own you know. But there was no way they'd have him back, I made a hell of a fuss about it. Not so much they didn't want him to go there, but the way they done it you know. So we have a big meeting with all the big noises and they said there's no way they'd have him back. They could put him residential, but I said no way will you put him residential, no way, and the only reason they had that meeting because – I didn't know at the time. My uncle was a councillor mind and he came with me because I showed him the letter and the only reason they had that meeting on condition that I wouldn't show the Press. Now I didn't know anything about that until after you see. I didn't want to get people into trouble, but that was the conditions on that meeting. They knew they had done wrong, so as I say, he was home from when he was 11 until he was 20.

QUESTION: When did you first start having contact with psychologists?

Mrs B. He must have been about 13 perhaps, I used to have him coming to the house and he was fantastic with him. He worked hard with him. But in the end he said I'm sorry you know – he had to give up, he really had to give up. He used to come once a week, once a fortnight to try and work with Malcolm here – he was ever so good, but he had to admit in the end you know, that there was no way he could do anything.

QUESTION: What did you used to do with Malcolm when you were home those 9 years?

Mrs B. I don't know! When I look back I don't know. My father was alive then and used to take him out a lot for me. My father used to watch him when I went shopping and he used to take him for walks, and take him for a run. Of course Bill was at work all day, he wasn't in until the evening. His behaviour was unbelievable – unbelievable. He used to have – the only way I can describe them is like brainstorms, that's the only way I can describe what he used to have. For no reason at all he'd go berserk and he'd go for me. If he could have got hold of me, he'd have killed me, he'd really go for me, you know, and thats when he used to smash windows with his hands, and doors, anything. And only once I thought I've got to do something with him and I thought if I can get him up into the bedroom and close the door on him. There was nothing he could harm there. I always make sure I've got things in front of my windows so he can't go to windows you know. Well, by the time I got him up and got him into that bedroom – I thought I was having a heart attack. I was lying on the landing because I couldn't breathe. He was screaming and yelling and banging in the bedroom. Eventually, he fell asleep and that's the first and only time he's ever slept during the day. He must have cried himself to sleep. It used to be terrible and it used to come on him like that. No reason at all.

QUESTION: When did you have the reinforced glass?

Mrs B. When he was having these attacks.

QUESTION: Even then you didn't think about having him put in a residential place.

Mrs B. No, no. I used to be sitting here crying many times and yet I still couldn't part with him. Maybe if I'd had other children I'd think well I've got to for their sake. You know. But with it being only him.

QUESTION: How did Malcolm affect your home life?

Mrs B. Well, we never had no home life. We could never go out together. Bill used to go out – he used to go out every night. He was alright as a husband but he wasn't a very happy person as well. He was never happy-go-lucky – and this on top of it as well then. Because we were married 5 years before I had Malcolm, and he just wouldn't accept that he was any different to any other child – you know. Just wouldn't accept it. I'd have to wait for him to be home at weekends so I could go shopping, and I used to say, I won't be long and it was fatal to say that. If I happened to call in my sisters on the way home and I was a bit longer – oh God – where have you been 'til now – you know. Do you know I've been so used to rushing about all my life, and this is true now, I can't slow down even now. It's only now I'm trying to slow down – I'm trying very hard to slow myself down – I'm trying to stop that for my own sake because I get very irritable – so I am trying. Like I say, Bill wouldn't go anywhere with us – he wouldn't even come for a walk. We never saw nobody.

QUESTION: What's life like with Malcolm now?

Mrs B. He used to get up at 4.00 am. This last month he's staying until about 6.00 or 6.30 am and that's great. Once he's awake we've got to get up – so we come down and he usually has his breakfast straight away. Then he has a bath, I clean his teeth, give him a shave, then I bring him back up and I dress him. And then weekends we usually go for a walk. He's dressed by about 7.30 am – its a long day. Between 7.30 and when the bus comes for the ATC I can't do anything, I can't leave him here. I can do the ironing – I put the iron here so I can watch him, but I leave everything then until he goes. During that time he doesn't do a lot – sometimes he'll have a little push at my furniture – he'll sit down mostly because he knows he's going. If I put his coat out, no matter what time it is, he knows he's going. He's home about 4.00 pm. He usually has tea then – straight away. Then he gets tired – he settles down and he just sits about. Then I give him a bit of supper and then he has a little wash, puts his pyjamas on and then once his pyjamas are on he really settles down for the night. He sits there and he's OK. He goes to bed about 7.30 pm, he cannot keep his eyes open. He normally sleeps right through. He used to be up at 2.00 am and 3.00 am. Weekends are very long and boring. He gets very agitated when he is home.

QUESTION: Is he still lashing out at you and scratching you?

Mrs B. He's been poorly the last 2 weeks so he's been OK but the last 2 or 3 months before he's been terrible – terrible. He'll do it for no reason at all – if I was walking past him he'd hit out at me for no reason at all. I know he does it when I've got to dress him or change his nappy or whatever but for no reason at all he was doing it, terrible. My mother has caught me crying many times these last few months because he hurts. I don't know. I had a psychologist here once and he said if you could ignore him when he is pinching or whatever, ignore it. Oh, I said, that's easier said than done because he hurts and you're bound to say stop it. But he didn't want me to say anything, to him and I said I'm sorry, that's not going to work, Because I've got to get it out of my system as well you know. Rather than smack him – I mean you've got to do something so I shout rather than smack him. You know how he can pinch and slap – its hard not to say anything to him. Well, for me its hard then – you know.

QUESTION: How would you like things to be different?

Mrs B. I can't see how they can be different. If you could say well – I don't know – I don't know how things can be any different for me. I mean I'm not prepared to put him residential. I've just got to learn to live with it.

QUESTION: What more help could people like myself give you?

Mrs B. I don't know Jan. I don't really. I'm more than grateful he goes to the centre.

QUESTION: Does he still go to the short-term care bungalow?

Mrs B. No. That's my fault. It's me. He's had about 3 overnight stays – the last one was April but I'm terrible. I worry terrible. I'm not saying he's not alright because he's fine. But – I don't know. I might try it again. They were wonderful, I'm not criticizing them, they were great. It's just me. I'm thinking what if he doesn't like it, what if he doesn't want to be there and then I think what if he thinks I've put him there and I'm not going back for him. You know? If he could talk and say mum, I don't want to go there, fair enough. But he can't say how he feels about being there – no. And yet, when I've gone in the morning he's quite happy. So much has happened these last 5 or 6 years – my father died so suddenly, then my grandmother then his dad dies, you know? In three years everything has gone – you know.

I did go on holiday this year my sister came down here to watch him and oh God! I went once before and I said never again, but its definitely never again – I was terrible. The first week I wasn't too bad – I think a week I could cope with but not two. We went to Greece – never again and yet he was fine. My sister said – you wouldn't believe how good he's been. He'd been ever so good for her – he wasn't even getting up until 8.00 am in the mornings. She said he was wonderful – no trouble at all for her. Never scratched or pinched her – nothing.

QUESTION: That must be quite hard for you to accept?

Mrs B. Yes, you know. I think, well, it's me you know. I must have cried all the way back on the plane. They must have thought I was crazy – I couldn't wait to get home and they'd brought him to the airport – I couldn't get to him quick enough. But he wasn't bothered! I know I'm over-possessive of him – I've got to do everything for him, its part of my life.

QUESTION: What are your hopes and fears for the future?

Mrs B. Not a lot of hopes I'm afraid. The only thing I'm dreading is I've got to die and leave him behind. I think about that a lot, that's the thing I can't live with – well I've got to live with it but that hurts the most. That's why they want me to take him to the short-term care bungalow and I know I'm being selfish. Death has got to come to us all – I've just made a will as a matter of fact because my sister will be his guardian and she said if anything happens to me that she will look after him for me. There again, there's not many years between my sister and myself, so you can't go by age can you. My greatest fear is leaving him behind. I've got two nieces and they love him and I know they'd have him but it's not fair – they've got their own lives. It's not fair. I've known what it is – I've had 20 years of it. No matter how good the staff are though – its not the same as family.

QUESTION: If you had three wishes for the future – what would they be?

Mrs B. Well I don't know. What do you think. Come on now Jan, what do you think? I wish my boy was alright, that's all.

Chapter Ten

EVALUATING COMMUNITY SERVICES

Social network analysis

PHILIP SEED

Social network analysis is a method developed by the Mental Handicap Research Team at the University of Aberdeen over the past 10 years; I shall first explain very briefly what it means, then illustrate its use with reference to the study of a patient discharged from hospital into the community, and finally outline an application of the techniques more generally to the discharge of patients from hospital. A full description of the methods is contained in *Applied Social Network Analysis* (Seed 1987a).

A network – any network – is a system of links between points. In social network analysis, the points represent significant people, places, or activities in daily living, and the lines represent the relationships between these points to the person we are studying, whom we will call the client. The purpose of the analysis is to provide answers to the question 'Which people, places, and activities are important in daily living?' This is an open-ended question which identifies informal as well as formal sources of support. It provides the context for evaluating specific services – for example, day-centres, domiciliary services, hospitals. It is based on the assumption that services which a client receives should be evaluated in the context of patterns of daily living.

This can be illustrated in terms of what we call 'information components' (Figure 10.1). In the top left we have the client's home base. In the bottom left we have a particular service or facility. The relationship between these two must be evaluated in the context of the significant people, places, and activities indicated on the right-hand side of the figure.

Amongst the information components at home we will need to know something about the client's social and health background.

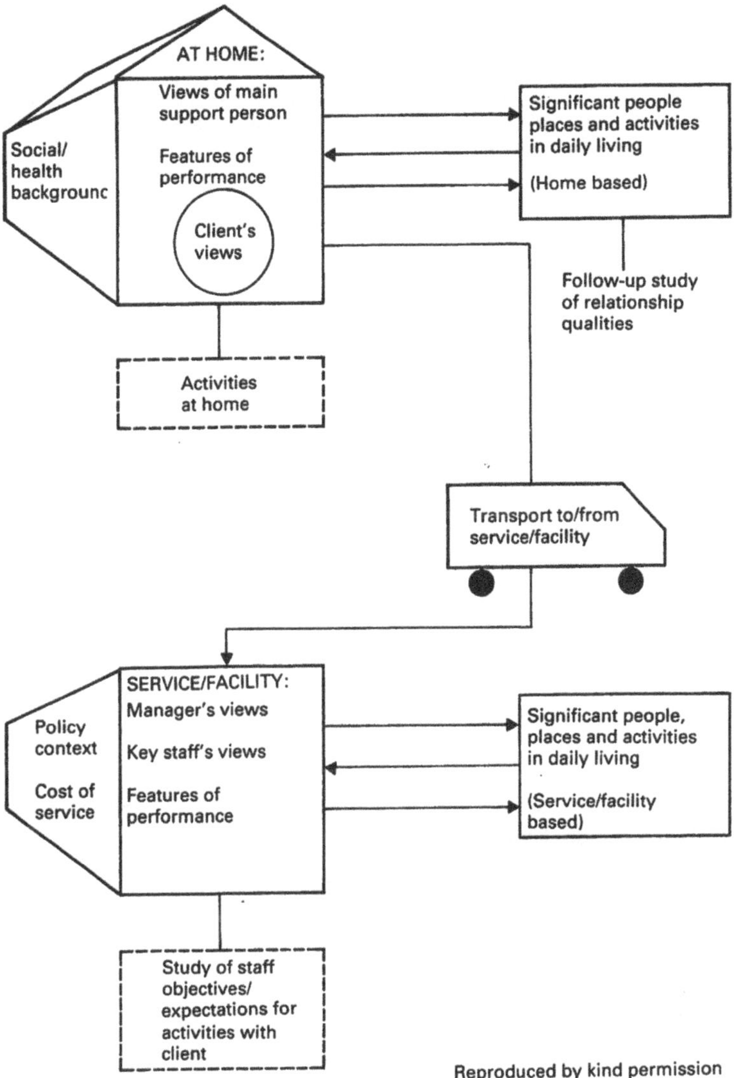

Reproduced by kind permission from Seed 1987a

Figure 10.1 Information components required

2. Wash, bath, and toilet

Yes, can accomplish adequately and without assistance/support	1	(22)
Yes, but to accomplish adequately requires assistance/support	2	
Possibly, but does not, in fact, do so	3	
No	4	
Other definite answers	9	
Not answered	0	

DETAILED COMMENT only if answer above coded 2-9

TASKS: Prepare for wash
Wash hands and face
Wash hair
Brush teeth
Get in and out of bath
Wash in bath
Get dried
Use toilet
Hold soap

ASSISTANCE NEEDED:

SUPPORT NEEDED:

COMMENT ON PROGRESS DURING PAST YEAR:

---

3. Eating and drinking

Yes, can accomplish adequately and without assistance/support	1	(23)
Yes, but to accomplish adequately requires assistance/support	2	
Possibly, but does not, in fact, do so	3	
No	4	
Other definite answers	9	
Not answered	0	

DETAILED COMMENT only if answer above coded 2-9

Figure 10.2 Example of self-management analysis

This includes information about the neighbourhood. We also need to know the views of the client himself or herself and the views of the 'main support person'. In the case of someone in hospital this might be a particular nursing officer. In the context of home it might be a parent or other relation.

Then we have what we call 'features of performance'. This is a description, rather than a check-list, of the client's ability to perform certain tasks at home. First, we are concerned with what we call 'self-management tasks'. These include looking after oneself in terms of dressing, washing, toilet, and so on. An example is shown in Figure 10.2. Second, we have what we call 'daily living tasks'. These include getting about independently, using money, preparing a simple meal, and so on. This is usually assessed by the main support person at home and, separately, at the service or facility with which we are concerned. It will be seen that we are also concerned with staff and management views and with the background to policy.

Moving across the figure to the important part, namely the people, places and activities that are important, these are studied by means of structured daily diaries. We have found that people like keeping diaries and the response rate is surprisingly good. Clients keep diaries in relation both to what happens at home and what happens at the facility they are attending. We ask each member of staff what their particular objective was on a particular day for each activity with a particular client (see Figure 10.3).

The analysis of all this information as a whole constitutes 'applied social network analysis'. A further aspect, following the completion of the diaries, is what we call a study of 'relationship qualities'. These are: qualities concerned with information and access to others; instrumental qualities (i.e. practical help and advice); what we call sentiment qualities concerned with feelings; and finally reciprocal qualities which relate to the client's opportunity to be helpful to others.

Let us now look at an example whom we will call Walter. (The following example is taken from one of two studies of patients leaving hospital in Seed 1987b). Walter was amongst a group of long-stay patients who left hospital 5 years ago. He moved first to staffed houses within a special 'village' run by a voluntary society. This rather unusual setting had previously been a well-known children's village. With the reduction of the numbers of children

Case number ☐☐☐☐ (1-4)

Staff number ☐☐ (7-8)

ACTIVITY AND CODE	IMPORTANCE CODE	STATEMENTS ABOUT OBJECTIVES AND CODE	PROBLEMS MENTIONED AND CODE
Activity code: ☐☐ (9-10) Activity status: ☐☐ (11)	(12)	**First objective:** Code: ☐☐☐☐ (13-16)	**First Problem:** Code: ☐☐ (18-19)
		Second ojective: Code: ☐☐☐☐ (23-26)	**Second Problem:** Code: ☐☐ (28-29)
		Third objective: Code: ☐☐☐☐ (33-36)	**Third Problem:** Code: ☐☐ (38-39)

Figure 10.3 Record and coding for staff statements relating to activities, objectives and problems

coming into care, it had changed and diversified. Providing stepping-stones for adults with mental handicaps leaving hospital was one of its new functions.

It is not clear how much preparation Walter had had before he left hospital. I was not involved in his life at that time, but from what he told me it seems to have been rather cursory. They were informed one day that they had been selected for the move and then were given some training for a few weeks to help them to be more independent. My involvement started two years after he had left hospital and he was followed through for a further 2 years during which time he moved on from this ex-children's village to live with his friend Susan in a council house in a town about 15 miles away.

Bearing in mind hair-raising accounts that one hears of long-stay ex-hospital patients being dumped on their own in the community, this must be an example of good practice in terms of community support. But what exactly does community support mean? David Brandon (Brandon 1986) has argued that a step-by-step approach of moving from hospital to hostel, hostel to group home, and finally group home to having one's own apartment or house is unsatisfactory. He calls the move from hospital to hostel 'trans-institutionalization'. Does the evidence of what happened to Walter justify such statements? To answer these two main questions, we need to look at the daily living patterns of Walter over a period of time and assess the restrictions, the opportunities, and the support he received from whatever source it came.

Walter was in the age-group 25–30 when he left hospital. He was relatively capable. He could undertake all of the self- management skills – for example, dressing, washing, eating, and so on – without any assistance or support. He could also perform all of our listed daily living skills except for one, namely he needed some assistance in understanding money.

This did not, however, inhibit him from going to shops. It was only suggested to us that he relied on the goodwill of shopkeepers not to short-change him.

Neither we nor Walter know much about his past. He had been in care since he was a baby and moved to a long-stay hospital when he grew up. It would seem fair to say that this would not happen today and that Walter represents the legacy of mistaken policies in the past.

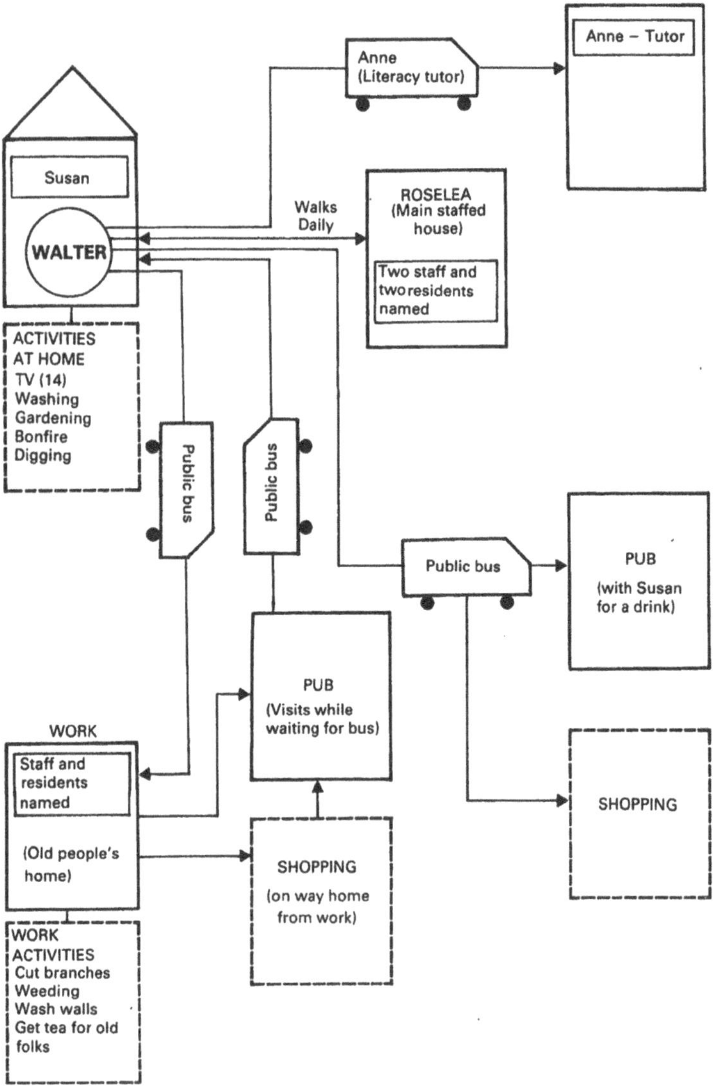

Figure 10.4 Walter – first monitored fortnight

By the time we met Walter in 1984 he had moved from the staffed house to an assisted cottage just outside the village. He shared this cottage with another ex-hospital patient called Susan. By this time Walter had attended an adult training centre (ATC) for two years. He had, however, been referred from the ATC to a new special project which is also well-known and which offers an alternative kind of day-care provision. Walter told us that he attended this special project to help him get out of the ATC and to help him to find a job. The move was highly successful and by the time we met Walter he had just started full-time as a gardener in the grounds of an old people's home.

Figure 10.4 shows the network drawing representing 14 days in Walter's life at this stage. It is based, so far as his home life is concerned, on diaries dictated by him to his key worker in the village. The record of activities at work is based on work sheets completed by him for the day-care project staff. Perhaps two aspects stand out from this network. The first is that Walter has friends and the second is that he has initiative in normalizing – if I can turn the noun into a verb – his own life. Notice that on the way home from work he goes shopping or visits the pub before catching the country bus to the village. While he has a network of friends within the village he also goes out with his friend Susan from the village. He also takes the bus at the weekend to another town to go shopping. At work he has contact not only with other staff but with some of the residents in the old folk's home. All of this may not seem too surprising except that there is one important point I have not yet mentioned. This is that Walter, apart from having a mild mental handicap, has a major speech impediment which at times can appear to be a severe disadvantage. In talking with him one is immediately impressed by his determination in overcoming it and in not allowing it to prevent him from doing anything he wants to do. We can also see from the network drawing that he is receiving personal adult literacy tuition. He is progressing well. Curiously, though, he is not receiving speech therapy and this was a point that was mentioned to us by his key worker.

I next visited Walter about ten months later. He now lived in a council house, still with Susan, and with a third person with a mental handicap who had not come from hospital but who had been encouraged to leave home and his parents. This third person in the group was not present and Walter and Susan explained to me that he did not always fit in so easily, partly because he had his mother on the doorstep. But Walter and Susan remained close friends. There was no suggestion that they were anything more than friends. They took it in turns to do household chores and share ideas for looking after the place, including, for example starting to do the garden.

This was an ordinary tenancy. They paid their rent monthly, and their only regular support, I was told, came from a social worker attached to a housing project. She was prepared to do such practical things as demonstrate cooking and taking them (on the first occasion) to the housing office so that they would know where it was that they had to pay the rent.

I asked Walter what worries or anxieties he had had. He mentioned three main worries. The first was how he would manage money; the second was how he would be able to cook; and the third was how he would get on with the neighbours and whether he would feel isolated. He explained that the social worker had helped with the first two of these problems and that the neighbours had turned out to be quite friendly. One had offered to be of assistance if needed. In general, however, Walter explained that the neighbours kept themselves to themselves and that he and Susan did the same. Meanwhile, Walter said he was still having his literacy tuition and still working at the same job. He said he enjoyed the summer more than the winter because there was less work to do in the winter time and he got bored. The house and garden were tidy and Walter showed me some of the house painting he had been doing. His stammering seemed much better. He told me he had been offered, or rather asked, if he wanted the services of a speech therapist and he had declined. He said he feared it could make him worse. I asked how he was coming on with his reading and whether he had reached the stage where he could say he enjoyed reading. He said he reads newspapers but his main hobby at home is listening to tapes and watching TV, apart from the gardening. I noticed that the house had a call-box telephone. I twice needed 10p change to use it myself and Walter had no difficulty in understanding that 2 x 5p = 10p. In general he seemed very relaxed. At one stage he told me some more details he had found out for the first time about his past. This is not the only case I have come across where people have only been able to find

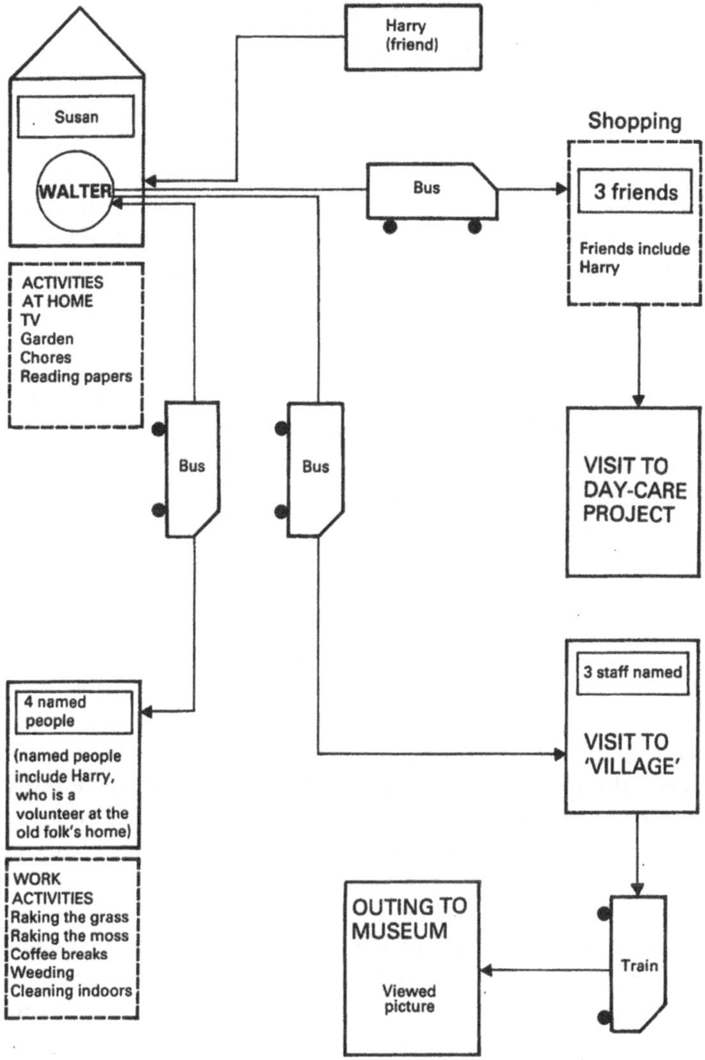

Figure 10.5 Walter – second monitored fortnight

out about their origins after they have left long-stay institutions.

My final visit to Walter was after another 6 months when we again asked him to keep diaries for us. This time Susan helped him write the diary entries. The network drawing for a fortnight is shown in Figure 10.5. The third person who shared the tenancy has now left and returned to his parents. He did not fit in and the move was premature, or perhaps he was wrongly placed. The relationship between Susan and Walter is still steady and platonic. Work is going well and we can see that Walter is still in touch with the day-care project through which he first obtained the job. Notice that he travels by bus and train – in fact, quite long distances – to meet friends and to go on outings. Notice also that one friend visits Walter at home. The house is situated on the very edge of town and this might be off-putting for some people to visit – although a bus takes you right to the door.

In terms of the principles of normalization, Walter has surely made it. What was this special day-centre project which did so much for him? (For another description of the project, see King's Fund 1985). The following are some of its key features which distinguish it from a traditional ATC. First, it has a group intake. Walter was one of eight who started at the same time. On the first day they meet together and mutual support is encouraged.

Second, they are accorded the status of potential 'workers' from the moment they arrive. Responsibilities for managing the group are shared – responsibilities which vary from who makes the tea to what they are going to do next.

Third, goals are set on the assumption that they will be realized within a limited time-span. Unlike a further education college course, the time-span is not precisely defined in advance but it is assumed to be about a year. The original object – successful in the case of Walter – was to find a job. In an area of about 30 per cent unemployment this is not easy and the goal has now been modified to include other forms of community activity.

Fourth, the centre is not a building, let alone a purpose-built one, where people attend regularly to undertake activities which are fixed from day to day, week to week, or year to year. The centre is a resource and those who attend go out to learn the skills they need in the community itself. Before finding work Walter had a series of placement experiences. Some of these could be within the same building since other things were going on in the building such as an old people's club. Here are some of Walter's comments at that time:

> The centre helps. If you've got any fault you can get over them. If you're stuck with anything you can get help. The day trips were useful. I learnt to travel back and forth. I had to learn numbers. But first I felt helpless.

Walter also received help from a very good key worker from the hostel he first attended and with whom he still maintains contact. He also had exceptional help from an adult literacy tutor. Finally, he had help from a social worker. All of these were components of successful care in the community, each of which was indispensable. Linked with this, resources and opportunities were available at the right time. He was able to get the tenancy of a house when he needed it. Finally, he was allowed to choose, for example, not to have a speech therapist, and his status as an adult was respected.

Applied social network analysis lends itself particularly well to assisting and monitoring the discharge of patients from long-stay hospitals. The following is an outline of nine stages which such an exercise entails.

(1) Establish basic information about all patients in the hospital relevant to a proposed programme of transfer to the community. For this purpose we would need the following information components: social background, features of performance in hospital, views of patient, views of main support person in hospital, views of next of kin in the community, current staff objectives.

(2) Identify which patients have priority. Who decides this? Do we look at facilities in the community, for example hostels, and then try to fill the places? Or do we look at the needs of our patients first and try to influence provision in the community in this light? If we are aiming for the latter then the next stage is:

(3) Survey of all intended developments in the community catchment area with a view to interrelating intended developments and the needs of patients.

(4) Network analysis by means of diaries at hospital. This includes the keeping of structured diaries and the follow-up of

What Happened Today:	List events or activities you can remember while you were at home (or hostel etc.)	Who were you with? If lots of people, name important people (If necessary, explain who they are)
Before going to the centre	Made my bed, helped Mum get breakfast	
During the day at the centre	Cooking, sewing, coloured picture	Arthur, Isobel, Janet, Mary, Margaret T.
During the evening or night	Watched TV Played tapes with Uncle George and my nephews. Then took dog for a walk to harbour	Uncle George, Aunty Mary, Mark, and Graham visited

Did you go out anywhere after returning from the Centre?

Places visited	Who with?	How did you travel?	Event or activity	Who else did you meet?
Harbour	Dog	Walk		No-one

Additional comments from person who assisted in completing diary:

Figure 10.6 Example of a diary format

relationship qualities. (An example of a diary format is shown in Figure 10.6.)

(5) Identify the client's preferences as far as placement options are concerned.

(6) Specific training/preparation for placement. The question arises as to how much can be 'taught' about independent living in a hospital setting.

(7) Is an intermediate move necessary? Perhaps the only argument justifying such a move is if it affords the client an environment in which real choice can be exercised.

(8) Monitoring. This involves network analysis by means of diaries at an interval after the move and subsequently.

(9) Aggregation of data for planning purposes.

POSTSCRIPT

I, or members of our team, are available for consultation in implementing the above or in any other aspect of making use of applied social network analysis. Contact Dr Philip Seed, Senior Research Fellow, The University of Aberdeen, Mental Handicap Research Team, Social Work Department, King's College, Old Aberdeen, AB9 2UB.

REFERENCES

Brandon, D. (1986) *Social Work Today*, 10 November, 16–18.

King's Fund (1985) *Towards a Normal Working Life*, London: King's Fund.

Seed, P. (1987a) *Applied Social Network Analysis – A Set of Tools for Social Services Research and Practice*, Tunbridge Wells: Costello.

——(ed.) (1987b) *Case Studies for Practice*, London: Jessica Kingsley.

Chapter Eleven

FROM COMMUNITIES TO NEIGHBOURHOODS

Evaluation

STEVE BALDWIN

DEFINITION AND TYPOLOGIES

Sociology

Examination of the evolution of the concept of neighbourhood to the present suggests that early formulations were often overinclusive and non-specific. One early definition (Park 1952) described neighbourhood as a 'natural area' involving: (a) a physically distinct geographical area, (b) a unique population, (c) a social system of rules/norms and patterns, and (d) distinctive life-styles and behaviours. The 'invasion – succession' model was developed from this sociological perspective, describing the process by which successive populations and social systems replaced each other. This focus on demography was complemented by a second sociological perspective, based on an analysis of physical environments. Social area analysts (for example, Greer 1962) viewed neighbourhoods on three main dimensions of social status, familism, and ethnicity. According to this second perspective, however, 'social areas' were not viewed as a physical entity of neighbourhood. 'Social areas' were instead defined by the presence of similar social characteristics.

This broad sociological focus on social variables has been refined in more recent years, and several attempts have been made to propose various typologies. Suttles (1972) proposed four types of neighbourhood, based on various levels of social organization: city face block (tenement), defended (a physically distinct residential system), community of limited liability, and expanded community of limited liability. More recently, Fischer (1976, 1982) has proposed social disorganization as a process by which to understand differences between neighbourhoods. These views of neighbourhoods as interaction systems provide an interesting framework to consider sociological perspectives. Moreover, this broad approach has demonstrated the need for fine-grain analysis of neighbourhoods.

Other attempts have been made to identify a typology of neighbourhoods (Warren, 1975; Warren and Warren 1977). Six 'types' have been proposed; (1) integral (cohesive, active, using internal resources); (2) parochial (classic, homogeneous, self-contained); (3) diffuse (static, selective, consensus); (4) stepping-stone (transient, activism, turnover); (5) transitory (dissensus, barriers, inaction); (6) anomic (individuated, unfocused, malleable).

Whilst invaluable as a set of observations based on considerable ethnographic fieldwork, the proposed system does not transcend the level of description of social events and physical structures. It does not offer a systematic framework based on empirical data. This failure to specify an adequate typology of neighbourhoods has coincided with a shift by sociologists to focus on dynamic models of neighbourhood change. Traditional explanations draw on the 'invasion – succession' model (Park 1952) and the 'life cycle' model (Hoover and Vernon 1959). The former is based on a resolution of conflict and resistance by locals and newcomers in a neighbourhood. The second model is based on a proposed five-stage change process of neighbourhoods; development, transition, down-grading, thinning out, and renewal. More recently, the two models have been used together, to describe neighbourhood movement through the life cycle as a series of invasion–succession cycles.

Contemporary sociological perspectives on neighbourhoods have synthesized several theoretical frameworks including demographic, ecological, socio-cultural, organizational, political, and economic perspectives (London 1980). In particular, the study of demographic and ecological perspectives has provided a bridge between the work of sociologists, and that of human geographers and economists. To date, however, the search for a typology of neighbourhoods, in the absence of strong methodologies, has yielded only social and physical variables. As a corollary, most sociological studies of neighbourhoods have been based on descriptive accounts, rather than based on a focus on evaluation.

Human geography

The study of neighbourhoods by human geographers has reflected some of the problems highlighted in sociological approaches. Specifically, some geographers have concluded that attempts to locate non-spatial, nominal classifications such as 'neighbourhoods' will be ultimately unproductive (for example, Kolars and Nystuen 1974). This perspective suggests that attempts to locate neighbourhoods on maps, using an abstract division of data, will have low utility in the investigation of interactions between people and places. In reality, the actual locations of nominal terms such as 'neighbourhood' may be as elusive as the end of the rainbow. The trend in this field has been to discard terms such as neighbourhood, in favour of more neutral constructs, such as 'locality'.

The study of human geography instead has extended the notion of 'locality' from the physical sciences. Several related ideas (for example, segregation, integration, central place theory) are based on the fundamental concept of functional associations between adjacent linear points. Thus, for example, the concept of 'segregation indices' relates to a calculation of the ratio of the population of a subgroup in an area, as a percentage of the total numbers in the whole group in that area. Clearly, the result of this calculation depends on both the size of the census unit, and the boundaries of that unit. When this example is applied in the context of the study 'neighbourhoods', it is immediately clear why many human geographers have opted to discard the term altogether.

The recent trend in this field parallels the 'paradigm shift' (Kuhn 1970) in the sociological study of neighbourhoods. Contemporary studies in the field are based on dynamic models of the interactions between people and places. The extension of 'central place theory', for example, has moved from a static to dynamic perspective of the process by which human populations tend to cluster around services sites. In this 'search for optimum sites', it may be possible to plan rationally where to locate both people, and the services they require.

Evidently, the methods of human geography have transcended the level of physical descriptions of people and places. The use of multifactorial analysis, including factor analysis and principal components analysis, have been applied to central place theory. This application of sophisticated statistical techniques is a trend towards a greater emphasis on evaluation. Progress in the field, however, is still restricted by long-running debates about the level of investigation and choices about units of analysis. Human geographers can use a range of conceptual 'filters' in their investigations of interactions between people and their environments. If 'coarse filters' are applied, not enough relevant information is generated; clots and clusters of data pass unnoticed. If 'fine filters' are applied, too many individual observations may be isolated. To date, progress in the field of human geography has been restricted by the search for 'medium filters'.

Environmental psychology

Historically, the perspectives of environmental psychology have been based on a behavioural model to explain interactions between people and places. In particular, the approach has been positivistic, with assumptions about human behaviour that tend to reduce the natural world to a featureless plane. The positivist approach assumes a social world of people not dissimilar to the physical world of objects. In addition, the positivist approach has encouraged beliefs in a set of value-neutral facts, and beliefs that actions and events are governed by 'natural laws'.

In recent years, there has been considerable criticism of this 'naïve determinism'. In particular, the adoption of natural science methodologies for the study of socio-spatial phenomena has been challenged (Lipman and Harris 1984). Other critics have suggested that traditional accounts of the interactions between people and places have been simplistic and repugnant (Harré and Secord 1972; Armistead 1974). According to this view, the study of neighbourhoods and physical space has been trivialized and oversimplified, using conceptually weak S–R models. In the context of the study of neighbourhoods, this contemporary critique of environmental psychology suggests that the adoption of a physical science model has produced a bias in the approach to the subject.

The study of neighbourhoods has been reduced to physical descriptions of surface manifestations, at the expense of a social understanding. This search for a set of irreducible principles to regulate human behaviour has produced an asocial, sterile, non-reflexive research practice (Lipman and Harris 1984).

This view of people as active agents in their physical environments has been endorsed by other investigators who have discarded the behavioural framework of environmental psychology. Instead, it has been proposed that people react and actively interpret their physical surroundings (for example, Rapoport 1982). According to this view, the affective component of individuals who inhabit neighbourhoods is determined by the *meaning* of those environments. This perspective takes account not only of the manifest function of physical surroundings, but also of the latent function; people develop images, beliefs, and ideals which they attach to their physical environments. This has often been noted in differences between meaning attached to environments by planners and architects, and users and residents: each group attaches different meanings to the same environment.

One major implication of this perspective for the study of neighbourhoods is to take account of the users' perceptions of their environments. If the meanings of physical environments are generated by personalization and possession (Rapoport 1982), there is a need to build in 'underdesign factors' into neighbourhood planning/evaluations.

Towards synthesis

Examination of sociological perspectives on the concept of neighbourhood brings the conclusion that the level of understanding and explanation has rarely exceeded that of descriptive accounts. Typically, these have been based either on an ethnographic approach (for example, Warren and Warren 1977) or on a more active involvement, in the method of participant-observation (for example, Henderson and Thomas 1980). Progress in the field beyond the level of description has been restricted by a perceived failure to specify an adequate typology of neighbourhoods.

In the field of human geography, there has been a trend towards substitution of non-spatial, nominal terms such as neighbourhood. Instead, natural science models have been adopted to study such relationships. In the search for precision and better specification, neighbourhood has been substituted by terms such as 'locality'. This model of physical reality is based on the relative position of people and places in three-dimensional space.

Contemporary developments in environmental psychology have produced a flux in the field. Traditional views of the relationships between people and places have been based on a deterministic, behavioural model. This mechanistic view of much of human behaviour as determined by environmental factors has received much criticism. Studies in the field have assisted in the refinement of the powerful technology of operant conditioning. Recent critics have, however, argued for the inclusion of mediating factors, such as understanding of the meaning of these environments for different people.

A synthesis of these three perspectives suggests that the search for the 'definitive' typology of neighbourhoods may be extremely difficult to find. As one observer has noted, 'there are no set of facts as elusive as neighbourhood facts' (Yin 1985).

It may even be counter-productive to prolong this search for a classification system. Evidently, any future attempts to produce such a system should transcend the level of previous subjective, descriptive accounts which lack any empirical base. Meanwhile, it is unsurprising that attempts at classification have produced much frustration: with so little agreement and so much confusion about definitions of neighbourhood, it is likely that these attempts will add little to an understanding of the concept.

This apparent disarray has prompted some observers to question the validity of the concept of neighbourhood. In particular, some critics have noted that neighbourhood is an ambiguous term, which does not have shared meaning amongst different people (for example, Allan and Higgins 1987). In particular, underlying assumptions about cohesiveness, size, unity, integration, and homogeneity in neighbourhoods have been challenged (Abrams 1986: Bulmer 1986).

It is highly appropriate to nurture the conditions for constructive dialogue and debate to examine underlying assumptions. It is inappropriate, however, to suggest abandonment of the concept altogether, in favour of the 'more neutral' term of locality, as some have proposed (for example, Allan and Higgins 1987). As noted, an examination of the field of human geography indicates that terms such as 'locality' are certainly not value-neutral. Moreover, the natural science origins in physics of such terms severely limit their applicability in the context of behavioural and social sciences.

Such criticism reveals that the concept of neighbourhood is at risk of devaluation. It is particularly revealing to observe the same criticisms of 'community' now applied to neighbourhood. This may have resulted from a fundamental failure to learn from previous errors of conceptualization and practice, with the concept of community. Thus, for example, it has been disconcerting to witness several recent attempts to specify the demographic size of neighbourhoods, in terms of minima and maxima (Henderson and Thomas 1980; Cumberledge 1986). Such attempts are doomed to failure.

Whilst, therefore, there are some unresolved questions about 'neighbourhood', it is a considerable improvement on the concept of community, which remains riddled with conceptual and practical problems. 'Community' has become unworkable as a way of understanding, planning, developing, or evaluating human services for client groups (Baldwin 1987). More than 30 years ago, ninety-four different definitions were identified (Hillery 1955). Overuse and abuse of terms such as so-called 'community care' and 'care in the community' have produced considerable confusion about their meaning. The current usage has become synonymous with 'non-hospital services', with no indication of location, type, range, quality, cost, or quantity. Such conceptual confusion has effectively set the conditions for non- evaluation of human services during the 1980s.

The challenge for neighbourhood studies

The current challenge for the future is to determine whether fact-gathering in neighbourhoods can be used as a process which is susceptible to empirical social science. The concept of neighbourhood may need to be defined differently; evidently the risk exists of conceptualizing 'neighbourhood' as a diminutive of community. This naïve reductionism should be resisted; evidently neighbourhood is also qualitatively different from traditional views about community. 'Neighbourhood' suggests social, physical, geographical, and cultural characteristics which relate to a specific phenomenon which is different from the unit of analysis of city, town, village, household, or individual.

Several obstacles to progress remain unresolved. In particular, it may be necessary to accept that no 'standard' definition of neighbourhood exists; possibly, the search for an all-purpose definition should be discontinued. Certainly, the current non-existence of this definition should not be a barrier to future investigations. A second barrier to progress relates to previous evaluation work which has been completed in the field: many studies report 'no-difference' or negative findings. This may have been the result of misapplication of inappropriate methodologies and technologies. Equally, however, it may be necessary to set the conditions whereby the reporting of negative findings becomes more acceptable (Yin 1985). In a general research climate which generates expectations of 'success' (Rossi and Freeman 1982), it may be necessary to alter the conditions to accept the negative findings of evaluation studies.

Other obstacles to progress relate to general difficulties of obtaining data for dependent variables in neighbourhood evaluations: the nature of the milieu is dynamic change, which produces inevitable problems for measurement and instrument validity. The lack of an adequate typology for neighbourhoods renders sampling techniques for comparative evaluation studies somewhat dubious; this has produced a trend to study individual neighbourhoods in isolation. These studies have relied on cross- sectional methods to measure changes over time. This has produced many single studies which do not specify adequate controls.

Further unresolved problems relate to units of analysis and levels of explanation in neighbourhood studies. 'Neighbourhood research' in practice may imply the study of small groups of people, which is clearly a separate phenomenon. The adequate specification of the focus for study will remain elusive as long as problems continue with definitions and typologies. In addition, it is often difficult to account adequately for external events when studying neighbourhoods; those forces are often remote and difficult to isolate.

These factors exert considerable influence on such investigations, to the extent that subsequent studies and evaluations often focus on individual neighbourhoods. This trend towards examination of isolated neighbourhoods has produced a reliance on single-case studies. In practice, many such investigations have been restricted to *post-hoc* analysis, or simplistic before-and-after studies (Yin 1985). The need remains to design robust, rigorous, comparative neighbourhood evaluations.

EVALUATION METHODOLOGIES

Planning an evaluation study

The best single justification for evaluation studies in neighbourhood work is the data yielded by such systematic investigation. In order to provide value for money to justify the additional expenditure, the study should be designed to produce valid and reliable evidence. Results of such investigations will provide the inputs for subsequent planning and policy-making. The optimum strategy to set the conditions for this outcome requires the use of scientific procedures to achieve maximum rigour in any particular situation. This will require a focus not only on outcome (ends), but also the process (means) by which this is achieved. Thus, the contents of the neighbourhood programme should not be restricted to statements about goals, but should also make statements about how these should be achieved.

Certain preconditions exist for testing neighbourhood programmes. In particular, the programme contents should be clearly specified, in order to be able to determine whether implementation has been successful (Rutman 1977). This will require detailed statements about desired goals and their intended effects. In practice, however, the 'real' programme goals may be obscure; hence, an exclusive focus on formally stated goals will be inadequate. Complementary monitoring of side-effects and unintended consequences is thus required. The rationale of the evaluation to the programme requires specification. This rationale is designed to address the fundamental question of evaluability assessment. It requires an analysis of decision-making systems and a clarification of the evaluation questions. In particular, it is imperative to know if the primary intended users have agreed the content, goals, and objectives of the neighbourhood programme. This approach to formative research evaluations requires an explicit commitment to feedback of results to the users following completion of the programme.

In order to examine the true purpose of individual neighbourhood programmes, it is necessary to clarify their stated goals and objectives. Many programmes will contain a hidden agenda and it is therefore essential to know the exact source of initiation of the evaluation (for example, Suchman 1972; Rutman 1977). In order to specify the relevant programme variables for measurement and evaluation, programme components should be correctly identified and articulated. This process of specification should enable similar identification of programme goals, and other possible intervening variables.

The rationale should outline how the programme can potentially accomplish goals. Despite this specification, however, the measures used to define the relative success of the programme will introduce considerable variation to the eventual outcome. In particular, the choice of indicators used to measure change will relate different ideological and theoretical positions. Recurrent problems of reliability and validity add to this variation. In order to reduce the effects of this variability, it is essential that the rationale contains explicit statements about the utilization of the findings of the evaluation. This may help to avoid the misapplication and reinterpretation of outcome data by groups with vested interests.

Designing an evaluation study

The single most salient criticism of so-called 'community care' and 'care in the community' programmes has been the failure to employ evaluation methodologies. The implementation of deinstitutionalization initiatives, in particular, has been characterized by non-evaluation as the standard (Praill and Baldwin 1988). Moreover, attempts at deinstitutionalization for a range of client groups, including elderly people, people with a mental handicap, and people with long-stay (rehabilitation) problems, have not been based on empirical evidence on efficacy or efficiency. Rather, such attempts have been based more often on moral, pragmatic, or political viewpoints. In particular, 'community care' has been used as an empty metaphorical counterpoint to 'non-hospital care'.

In a dominant ethos where evaluation has been viewed as a luxurious afterthought to the design and implementation of human services, it has been difficult to modify attitudes and behaviour to favour such initiatives. In particular, it has been difficult to integrate the concept of evaluation at the design stage.

This has been partly due to a lack of an agreement about what constitutes a strong evaluation methodology. To date, social science methods have been adopted in human services evaluations: in a field with a relatively short history and dubious pedigree, the rules of data collection have not yet been determined, and remain unclear. As yet, consensus about research designs has not been achieved.

The evaluation of neighbourhood services has produced several characteristic problems, which relate to initial decisions about design. Specifically, the design elements required for comparisons and statistical analysis have created methodological problems. Thus, for example, the identification of appropriate control groups, randomization of subjects/interventions, and the generation of sufficient data points to allow the meaningful application of statistical procedures – all present particular problems for the evaluation of neighbourhood services. Such elements, however, are fundamental to a robust design, (Fitz-Gibbon and Morris 1987) and will require resolution to permit the development of more adequate methodologies for neighbourhood evaluations.

A further problem for the rational implementation of neighbourhood services has been a prevailing view that has marginalized evaluation attempts as an activity unrelated to service provision itself (Patton 1982). One aim of neighbourhood services, therefore, should be to create a subsequent climate in which evaluation initiatives become an explicit goal of service provision. In a context in which statutory funding agencies often view the fundamental aim of service provision as the guarantee of 'minimum standards', it is potentially threatening to generate data which indicate 'negative' outcomes. The design of neighbourhood evaluations therefore should attend specifically to questions about the audience for subsequent reports, and utilization of findings.

Designs for neighbourhood evaluations

Four types of research design have produced promising results in the evaluation of neighbourhood services:

(1) True Control Group, pre-test post-test
(2) Non-Equivalent Control Group, pre-test post-test

(3) Single Group Time Series
(4) Time Series with Non-Equivalent Control

Time control group, pre-test post-test

The classical design requires random assignment of subjects to two groups, E and C. The design requires that Group E receives Programme X. Group C, meanwhile, receives no programme, or an alternative programme, Y. Providing that pretest scores show Groups E and C to be equivalent, differences at post-test can be attributed to Programme X.

This is a powerful design, which permits direct comparisons of programmes in neighbourhoods. Frequent problems of true randomization, however, can make implementation of this design difficult in neighbourhood evaluations.

Non-Equivalent control group, pre-test post-test

This design requires the formation of a comparison Group C, which is similar to the experimental Group E. These groups, however, are not formed by random assignment. The formation of Group C requires the identification of a group which is as similar as possible to E. Group E receives Programme X, whilst C receives no programme, or an alternative programme. Information should be collected about ways in which Groups E and C are similar and different at pre-test. If it can be demonstrated that E and C are approximately equivalent, it is possible to attribute differences at post-test to Programme X.

This design is less powerful than the previous one; it is more practical, however, for neighbourhood evaluations. In practice, it is difficult to achieve true randomization, whether by neighbourhoods, interventions or clients. This design offers a pragmatic solution to the requirements of statistical analysis.

Single group time series

This design does not permit comparisons between neighbourhoods; rather, it is applied to studies of individual neighbourhoods. It requires the collection of data with test measures at regular intervals prior to the implementation of Programme X. This experimental Group, E, can be formed either by repeated administration of the test measures to the same group over time, or to a succession of groups. The test measures are then repeated during Programme X. Finally, these measures are repeated at regular intervals after completion of Programme X. Examination of time series graphs plotted from test measures allow extrapolation of trends in the data. Elimination of other explanations for subsequent changes in levels of the test measures allows the conclusion that these changes were a result of Programme X.

This design offers an ideal method of analysis for the evaluation of programmes in individual neighbourhoods. Whilst it does not allow comparisons between different studies, it is a useful design using a neighbourhood as its own control

Time series with non-equivalent control

This is an extension of the previous design, with the addition of a comparison group. Having identified the E group, another Group, C, should be located which is as similar as possible to E. The programme of Group C can be designated Programme C. Test measures are then collected for both Groups E and C at regular intervals. These measures are repeated during the implementation of programmes E and C. Following completion of the programmes, the test measures continue at the same regular intervals. Differences between E and C which cannot be explained by other factors/events can be attributed to Programme E.

This design offers many possibilities for neighbourhood evaluations. It can be applied both to investigate comparisons between neighbourhoods, and also to examine the effects of different interventions within the same neighbourhood.

The complexity of neighbourhood evaluation

These quasi-experimental designs offer a range of applications in field settings (Campbell and Stanley 1966; Campbell 1969; Cook and Campbell 1976, 1979). A firm commitment to principles of design and implementation has assisted their application in the USA in some neighbourhood evaluations (for example, Rossi and Freeman 1982). Examination of recent studies in the UK, however, indicates that many neighbourhood projects have not been subject to formal evaluations. Much of this work in neighbourhoods has been based on flimsy methodology and very weak designs, such as before-and-after studies (for example, Baldwin 1986; Baldwin and

Baser 1986); descriptive demographic surveys (for example, Cunningham et al. 1985); and after-only designs (for example, Bayley and Tennant 1985; Abrams 1978, 1980).

It has been difficult to achieve a true commitment to evaluation principles in the applied settings of neighbourhoods. Thus, whilst social science methods have offered a promising range of evaluation technology, much neighbourhood work has been conducted in the absence of any formal evaluation. This may be due partly to a historical phenomenon; traditionally, social workers and community workers often have been the most frequently represented professional groups involved in neighbourhood work. These groups are not renowned for a commitment to evaluation research. Much sociological enquiry has been conducted using a method of participant-observation (Henderson and Thomas 1980; Yin 1985) and ethnographic study (Warren and Warren 1977).

In practice, a rational balance between 'objective' and 'subjective' data has been extremely elusive in the field of neighbourhood work. Studies which have relied on soft, impressionistic accounts of interventions have been unconvincing; equally, studies which have relied solely on 'products', at the expense of consideration of 'process' variables, have sometimes been overcommitted to an objective, 'hard-nosed' approach to evaluation. Accurate performance measures are required, which generate relevant information about intervention effects, with respect to the original programme goals. This explicit commitment to measurement of initial and current performance levels allows rational decision-making; it requires, however, a prerequisite of clear, accurate, and precise programme objectives and goals (Spiegel 1977).

The complexity of neighbourhood evaluations also requires an appreciation of the subject to 'ownership'. Frequently, residents and users of services in neighbourhoods have been excluded in design and implementation (Hester 1975). Similarly, evaluation initiatives frequently have not been initiated as a result of consumer requests (Patton 1982). An appreciation of the political reality of evaluation studies requires the recognition that the use of information and data is not value-free.

Participation and involvement of consumers in design should meet a least four minimum requirements: (1) consumers should 'own' it; (2) an adequate sampling of users should occur; (3) a commitment to gradualism and impermanence; and (4) the use of a satisfactory medium to represent accurately the final design (Kaplan 1978). True consumer involvement as eventual 'stakeholders' (Patton 1981, 1982) should be a prerequisite for all neighbourhood evaluations.

Improving neighbourhood evaluations

The single most important reason to insist on evaluation in neighbourhood work is to be able to distinguish between useful current programmes and ineffective or inefficient programmes. Given appropriate design and implementation, evaluation data should inform about the nature and scope of problems, and which programmes and interventions are best matched to particular populations. Such data should also be informative about costs-benefits and effectiveness. This systematic use of social- research procedures is more than an application of methods: given a sound rationale, evaluation should become an integral part of social policy and public administration. Whilst it is apparent that human services and statutory government agencies operate according to different sets of norms, the results of local neighbourhood evaluations should form an essential input to the complex mosaic of national service-provision.

Evaluation initiatives should therefore exert a major influence on subsequent improvements to service delivery, as well as providing an explicit mechanism for accountability. Decisions about continuation, expansion, or curtailment of service components should be linked to feedback from evaluation questions. The legitimation for individual programmes (and subsequent policy) should be linked to estimates of percentages of successful implementation and target completion. Neighbourhood evaluations should have specific consequences for subsequent features of design, implementation, timeliness, and staffing (Rossi and Freeman 1982). In field settings, however, it has been difficult to consistently produce timely and unambiguous findings with high reliability and validity. In reality, most evaluation initiatives are likely to be a mid-point between what is ideal, and what is feasible.

Future improvements to neighbourhood evaluations may

require the recognition that traditional social science research designs ultimately may have limited applicability. Other models from economics, history, and even political science may offer alternative frameworks for neighbourhood evaluations. Certainly, no single research model exists for such evaluations, and choice of design depends on the local setting and constraints. Despite these variations, however, the fundamental question in neighbourhood evaluations remains: has this programme improved conditions for users /clients in this neighbourhood?

Several unresolved problems relate to this question. First, there is the collective nature of the unit of analysis of 'neighbourhood', which poses major problems for purposes of comparison. Second, it is apparent that interventions work unevenly across the whole unit: 'user/client behaviour' cannot be readily translated into a 'neighbourhood effect'. Third, the nature of political and administrative reality produces difficulty for implementation: in practice, interventions become staggered over time, which contaminates subsequent data collection. Fourth, it is extremely difficult to obtain meaningful, accurate, reliable, and valid test measures. Fifth, the application of traditional research designs, in particular the need for randomization and control groups, has been very elusive. Sixth, it has frequently been an uphill struggle to persuade management and administration to provide adequate funding for robust evaluations.

There are evidently no immediate solutions to all these questions. The increasing recognition of the need to involve users / clients is, however, a welcome and overdue shift in perspective. The early involvement of users as 'stakeholders' (Patton 1981, 1982) in evaluation research initiatives has helped to resolve some problems of ethics, implementation, and accountability. The single outstanding task within neighbourhood work remains to shift the dominant ethos of evaluation from 'expensive luxury item' to 'essential prerequisite'.

REFERENCES

Abrams, P (1978) 'Neighbourhood care and social policy: a research perspective', Berkhamstead, Herts: The Volunteer Centre.

——(1980) 'Social change, social networks and neighbourhood care', *Social Work Service*, 22 February: 12–23.

——(1986) *Patterns of Neighbourhood Care: Ten Case Studies in Their Social*

Contexts, Durham: Rowntree Research Unit, University of Durham.
Allan, G. and Higgins, J. (1987) 'A sentimental notion?' *Community Outlook*, June: 30–1.
Armistead, N. (1974) 'Introduction', in N. Armistead (ed.) *Reconstructing Social Psychology*, Harmondsworth: Penguin.
Baldwin, S. (1986) 'Systems in transition: the first 100 elderly people', *International Journal of Rehabilitation Research* 9: 139–48.
——(1987) 'From communities to neighbourhoods – I', *Disability, Handicap and Society* 2 (1): 41–59.
—— and Baser, C. (1986) 'The Emperor's new clothes', *Community Outlook*, February: 19–21.
Bayley, M. and Tennant, A. (1985) 'Interservice collaborations at the very local level: some findings from the Dinnington Project', *Research Policy and Planning* 2(2): 9–13.
Bulmer, M. (1986) *Neighbours: The Work of Philip Abrams*, Cambridge: Cambridge University Press.
Campbell, D. T. (1969) 'Reforms as experiments', *American Psychologist* 24 (April): 409–29.
——and Stanley, J. C. (1966) *Experimental and Quasi-Experimental Designs for Research*, Stokie, Illinois: Rand McNally.
Cook T. D. and Campbell, D. T. (1976) 'The design and conduct of quasi-experiments and true experiments in field settings', in M. B. Dunnette (ed.) *Handbook of Industrial and Organisational Research*, Stokie, Illinois: Rand McNally.
——(1979) *Quasi-experimental Design and Analysis Issues for Field Settings*, Stokie, Illinois: Rand McNally.
Cumberledge, J. (1986) *Neighbourhood Nursing – a Focus for Care*, London: HMSO.
Cunningham, B., Evans, J., and McNaughton, A. (1985) 'Petersfield resources and services for people with a mental handicap', unpublished paper, Portsmouth Health Authority.
Fischer, C. S. (1976) *The Urban Experience*, New York: Harcourt Bruce Jovanovich.
——(1982) *To Dwell Among Friends*, Chicago: University of Chicago Press.
Fitz-Gibbon, C. T. and Morris, L. L. (1987) *How to Design a Program Evaluation*, 2nd edn, Beverly Hills, CA: Sage.
Greer, S. (1962) *The Emerging City: Myth and Reality*, New York: Free Press.
Harré, R. and Secord, P. F. (1972) *The Explanation of Social Behaviour*, Oxford: Basil Blackwell.
Henderson, P. and Thomas, D. L. (1980) *Skills in Neighbourhood Work*, London: Allen & Unwin.
Hester, R. T. (1975) *The Neighbourhood Space*, Stroudsburg, PA: Bowden Hutchison Ross.
Hillery, G. A. (1955) 'Definitions of community: areas of agreement', *Rural Sociology* 20 (June): 11.
Hoover, E. M. and Vernon, R. (1959) *Anatomy of a Metropolis*, Cambridge, MA: Harvard University Press.

Kaplan, R. (1978) 'Participation in environmental design; some considerations and a case study', in S. Kaplan and R. Kaplan (eds) *Humanscope: Environments for People*, North Scituate, MA: Duxbury Press.
Kolars, J. F. and Nystuen, J. D. (1974) *Human Geography: Spatial Design in World Society*, New York: McGraw Hill.
Kuhn, T. S. (1970) *The Structure of Scientific Revolutions*, Chicago: University of Chicago Press.
Lipman, A, and Harris, H. (1984) 'Environmental psychology – a sterile research enterprise?' *Built Environment* 6(1): 68–74.
London, B. (1980) 'Gentrifications and urban reinvasion: some preliminary definitional and theoretical considerations', in S. B. Laska and D. Spain, (eds) *Back to the City*, New York: Pergamon Press.
Park, R. A. (1952) *Human Communities*, Illinois: Glencoe.
Patton, M. Q. (1981) *Creative Evaluations*, Beverly Hills, CA: Sage.
——(1982) *Practical Evaluation*, Beverly Hills, CA: Sage.
Praill, T. and Baldwin, S. (1988) 'Beyond hero innovations: real change in unreal systems', *Behavioural Psychotherapy* 16: 1–14.
Rapoport, A. (1982) *The Meaning of the Built Environment: A Nonverbal Communication Approach*, Beverly Hills, CA: Sage.
Rossi, P. H. and Freeman, H. E. (1982) *Evaluation: A Systematic Approach*, 2nd edn, Beverly Hills, CA: Sage.
Rutman, L. (1977) 'Planning an evaluation study, in L. Rutman (ed.) *Evaluation Research Methods*, Beverly Hills, CA: Sage.
Spiegel, H. B. C. (1977) 'Evaluating program results', in H. W. Hallman (ed.) *The Organisation and Operation of Neighbourhood Councils: A Practical Guide*, New York: Praeger.
Suchman, E. (1972) 'Action for what? A critique of evaluative research', in C. H. Weiss (ed.) *Evaluating Action Programmes*, Boston, MA: Allyn & Bacon.
Suttles, G. (1972) *The Social Construction of Communities*, Chicago: University of Chicago Press.
Warren, D. (1975) *Black Neighbourhoods: An Assessment of Community Power*, Ann Arbor: University of Michigan Press.
Warren, R. B. and Warren, D. I. (1977) *The Neighbourhood Organizer's Handbook*, Notre Dame: The University of Notre Dame Press.
Yin, R. K. (1985) *Conserving America's Neighbourhoods*, New York: Plenum

Chapter Twelve

EVALUATION OF COMMUNITY SERVICES

A local example

ANNETTE HAMES

The aim of this chapter is to present basic ideas in order to help others get started on evaluative research. It will not be concerned with a purely academic approach to evaluation, with statistical significance, control groups, and so on. Rather, it will present some ideas on how the reader can carry out a study and do something that is going to be useful. In particular, it will concentrate on how to identify and specify the aims of the research, and will look at what one has to do in order to achieve these aims.

To start at square one, therefore, what is a study for? First of all it is to prove a point. What is the point? As someone pointed out recently, is it just to prove that 'I am clever'? 'I can write papers'? Well, sometimes there is a more useful point to be made. Second, why undertake the study, and finally, how? This chapter will follow through these points, one by one, and then follow the same process in describing a local study.

If someone is about to undertake an evaluative study, the first question is: *what* is the point they want to prove? What are the aims? In other words, is there a hypothesis? It cannot be said that there is not a hypothesis, as researchers must have some idea when setting out their questions, what they are after. It would be naïve to say that one did not know what to expect from a study. One has to acknowledge that there are some expectations and that these in turn will affect the way in which the study is conducted and questions asked. Also, would anyone have the luxury of being allowed the time to study something, having no idea what he or she was likely to find? There often is a hypothesis there. So what is the point to be made? What is the aim of the study?

There are four types of aims:

(1) that a service is doing what clients/families want it to do;
(2) that a service is doing what it says it is doing, and what people paying for it think it is doing;
(3) that a service is 'better' than another service;
(4) that a service is good value for money.

These aims are all quite distinct and require different approaches, and demand different questions to be asked. Of course it may be the case that a study intends answering more than one of these questions, but one has to be clear to start off with about what the intention is, what point is to be made. Let us start with the first one, and really the most important question: is a service doing what clients/families want it to do?

This is the sort of question that is frequently forgotten. Professionals get involved in identifying what they believe people ought to be doing, how they ought to be behaving, particularly when working with people who cannot easily make their own needs clear, for example people with a severe mental handicap. When working with that group of people, it is too easy to determine what one thinks they want, and believe that they want the same as the professional. So it is a valid question: is a service doing what clients/families want it to do? It might be doing exactly what the professional thinks it should be doing, but something quite different to what clients and families think it should be doing!

What is the second point to consider? Is a service doing what it says it is doing – that is, is it doing what the people who are paying for it think it is doing? So what is needed? There needs to be somewhere where it is stated what the service is doing, i.e. an operational policy or philosophy of the service. If there is not an operational policy, maybe the service is guided by some principles from an influential document – for example the King's Fund Document, *An Ordinary Life* (1980) – and this can be used to describe what the service should be doing.

A third question is: is a service 'better' than another service? But what is a 'better' service, or 'better' life? Who is going to define it? How is it going to be measured? Is this better for professionals or better for others? Best for me, or best for the person who is older than me, or a person who has been in hospital all her life? Better for individuals or better for society? These are philosophical and political questions, not research questions, and there is a moral aspect embedded here. In Victorian times and the heyday of the Bethlam Hospital, it was felt to be better to keep people with mental illness and mental handicap (there was no distinction) and those who had illegitimate children (probably thought to be the same) far away from others, but in an environment specifically tailored to their needs. It was thought that these people were sexually over-active, bred like rabbits, and therefore it was 'better' that they should be segregated. Now the view is that community care is best, that people who were previously segregated and locked away should be allowed to live with their family and friends, in as normal an environment as possible, with additional specialized services, in order to encourage development of their full potential – which, it is argued, will be more likely to develop in a normal environment. Some people will still disagree, however, about whether it is 'better' to integrate children in school. Is it 'better' for them to have the confidence of knowing that they are the cleverest in a special school, or the confidence of knowing that they are attending a normal school like all their peers, even if they find it difficult? What is needed is to define exactly what is meant by 'better', which are the indicators which are important for those doing the study and for the people who are being studied, then measure whether there are more or less of these in the services which are to be compared. Now this is a research question!

Though if one believes that one service is 'bad' in some way, does it have any meaning to say that another service is 'better' than one which is considered to be 'bad'? So what if a community service is 'better' on some indices than a hospital service? That might mean nothing. It might not be much better and it is not uncommon to hear of 'bad' community services, for example people from psychiatric hospitals being discharged to seedy hotels and poor-quality seaside guest- houses.

The fourth question is: is it good value for money? – usually not explicit but probably implicit, particularly if the evaluation is being completed for the people who are responsible for paying for the service. But of course, it is an impossible question to be answered. How on earth does one put a price on quality of life? This has been attempted by research by Professor Williams (Williams 1986) from York, where he describes 'Qualies', which refer to quality years.

These are ways of trying to estimate the number of healthy and useful years one has after various health procedures. The way that one could go about estimating whether a service is good value for money would be to start by stating the objectives of a good-quality community service, i.e. quality objectives.

The next question to be asked after *what* is the point to be proved is *why* prove it? Here one is concerned with what action will follow the study and whether there is a commitment to change – though, of course, there does not have to be change. It could be that the intention of the study is that 'this is good, therefore it should remain pretty much the same', but it may be the intention to show that 'this could be better, therefore things should change'. If the intention is that change is necessary, at what level will it be recommended that change should occur – at the level of the individual, the service, or society? If, for example, the evaluation asked the question 'can this house support these very handicapped/dependent residents' and the finding was that there were problems in the house, would the intended change be at the level of the individual – that the residents are too dependent and, therefore, less dependent people should move in; at the level of the service – that there are not enough staff in the house and external staff support, and therefore this should be increased; or at the level of society – that the local community was not prepared for these very dependent people moving into their locality and that the service should consider some form of community education? Those asking for the information, those carrying out the study and those receiving the information must be clear and agree about how change is most likely to be achieved.

Something which has permeated this chapter so far is that there is a moral issue underlying all of this. One has to agree with the moral underpinning in order to carry out an evaluation effectively. In order to show that one service, in some way or ways, is better than another, is there agreement on the definition of 'better'? In order to measure whether a service is good value for money, does one believe in the quality objectives set, and have no short-cuts been made? If change is to be recommended, is there agreement with the level at which it is recommended that change be made? In the past, many more studies described changing individuals, especially changing their behaviour, particularly if they did not fit in. Following this there was an understanding that frequently, difficulties arose with individuals because of poor staffing and so it was the service which needed to change. Now there is more awareness of a need for community education. Much public outcry about community facilities for people discharged from hospital is based on public ignorance. Perhaps there might be less outcry if there was better preparation and community education. So one has to be certain about the level at which one believes change is effective.

So from *what* is the point, through *why* do the study, leads to *how* to undertake the study? The four types of evaluation pinpointed initially will be returned to and descriptions of how one might go ahead with each of these will be described using examples from a number of studies.

The first type of evaluation mentioned was: is the study doing what clients/families want it to do? Well, if someone wanted to buy a house, could someone else tell them what would be the best house to buy? Of course not. One person does not necessarily know what is best for another. So if the aim of the study is to find out whether a service is doing what clients/families want it to do, then one has to ask them. Even though the researcher might think that frequently getting out to evening activities is a positive about a community house, someone who lives there and has spent his or her life being pushed out of a ward to hospital discos might be glad of the opportunity to stay in alone and watch television.

In fact it is not only in service evaluation that clients' views are frequently not gained, but even in service provision clients are not consulted. How often are families involved in planning and the purchasing of houses and determining house philosophy? Very rarely!

Thus, if one is to ask clients and their families what service they want and whether the service meets their needs, and if clients are able to speak for themselves, they could be asked directly. If the stated aim of the service is to meet family needs, and adult clients do not object, their families could be asked too. For a service which aims to meet the needs of families, where the clients are children or adults who have difficulty in speaking for themselves, once again one could ask the families. Or maybe they have advocates who could speak on their behalf. The presumption here is that local services are to meet both the needs of clients and their families, in order that people are not cut off from their families.

Thus, if one is going to ask people if a service is doing what they think it ought to be doing, and the people are happy there, what areas should be asked about? Studies have related happiness to good health, enjoyable work, simplicity, stimulation, friendship, and affection.

Some technical points should be mentioned, however. If one is going to speak to people who are not used to answering questions, who have perhaps not had many choices in their lives, and who are possibly unsure about why they are being asked questions anyway, one has to beware of people's tendencies in these situations to answer 'yes' all the time. Some people have tried getting around this problem by asking 'either/or' questions, but these tend to be slightly harder to answer, and subsequently it has been found that there is a tendency to agree to the second option mentioned. What can be done is to ask questions where sometimes someone has to answer 'yes' to give a positive response, and sometimes 'no'. However, beware of the double-negative – 'was it not that you didn't like it when she didn't tell you that you weren't supposed to do it?'! (Heal and Chadsey-Rusch (1985) give an example of questionnaire design).

Of course, it may feel that by asking structured questions, one is still determining what people say. However, it is certainly easier to start off with structured questions rather than just asking 'what do you think of this place?'. A structured questionnaire also makes it easier to summarize and report back on one's findings. One could start with a questionnaire and when the interviewee has opened up a little, go on to more open-ended questions and general discussion.

Studies which have asked people what they think about the place they are living in, and have asked them to compare it with living in a hospital, have come up with the following sorts of responses. The freedom of a small, community-based facility has been found to be the main bonus. This compares with the restrictions people have felt whilst living in a hospital environment, particularly by authority and rules imposed by the hospital staff. Studies have also found that people generally do not mind being involved in domestic chores, particularly so if these have been denied them before (Passfield 1983).

The next question at the beginning was: is the service doing what it says it is doing, i.e. what those who are paying for it think it is doing? As stated earlier, is there an operational policy or philosophy of the service? If there is not an operational policy drawn up, then could one refer to relevant published documentation? For services for people with a mental handicap, for example, one could refer to the King's Fund Document *An Ordinary Life* (1980); for elderly people, the King's Fund Document *Living Well into Old Age* (1986); and people with psychiatric difficulties, again a King's Fund Document, *A Checklist of 20 Questions: Creating Local Psychiatric Services* (1983).

When looking through an operational policy, it may be that some parts are much easier to operationalize than others. Thus for example, the philosophy section will always be more difficult. One needs a philosophy, however, and it may be that questions which are asked in the evaluation are based upon other sections of the operational policy, using the philosophy section to frame the questions and answers for which one is looking.

So on to the third question: is a service 'better' than another service? It is important to remember to define exactly what is meant by 'better'. Then there is the practical point of choosing the indices carefully in order to determine which is 'better'. If the indices are biased, of course, one can prove that one service is 'better' than another. Let us take two individuals. Say it had been determined that the definition of 'better' was 'fitter'. Now which one of these two is the fitter? One might be better at arm wrestling, the other might be faster over a half marathon! Both are fit, but which one turns out to be the fitter will depend upon the indices chosen. In the study of staffed houses for young people, to be described later, of course the young people had more frequent contact with their families than they had previously. They had moved to houses half a mile away from their families, whereas the hospital where they lived previously was miles away, and most of the parents did not have transport. Of course the children visited community facilities more often because these were around the corner and no longer a mile walk into town. Of course they got more involved in kitchen tasks, because food was cooked in the house and not brought in from another ward.

The final question is whether a service is good value for money. As described earlier, here one needs to define quality objectives. Thus, for example, a good-quality placement could mean that everyone has their own bedroom; that people can have three cooked meals a day; that there are always enough staff on duty so that residents, who need staff accompaniment, do not have to go out in large groups; and that the staff have enough time, apart from doing domestic and routine duties, to spend time with people. Of course, it would be cheaper to share bedrooms, only have toast for breakfast, and provide a minimum of staff so that routine tasks can be completed, but no social interaction takes place. But then, if quality objectives are not set, of course the quality of life will become worse as money is saved. Setting the objectives of a good-quality service and then costing these seems to be the way to start to establish whether the service is good value for money.

Included with *how* is one going to do the evaluation are – who to involve and how to feed back the information? Starting with who is involved, if one requires commitment then one has to involve others, and there are three groups here: those requesting information, those collecting information, and those receiving information. Those involved in requesting the information ought to take part, and they need to define exactly what they want, otherwise they are bound to complain afterwards that something has been left out. 'Could you just go back to the beginning again, and collect just that one piece of information over the last 5 years'!

Those involved in collecting the information need to be involved, including their managers as well, of course. The greater the involvement, the greater the commitment and, hopefully, the faster things get done! Finally, those receiving the information are added as a separate group as they are not necessarily one and the same as the group of people who request the information. It may be that the fruits of hard labour are to be widely spread, but one has to be sure that the information collected is of interest and use to all parties concerned.

Of course, the researcher has to ask whether he or she is the best person to be involved anyway! Apart from the question of whether one knows enough about research methodology, has got enough time, or is good at writing reports, who is going to make most impact in carrying out the research and effecting change subsequently? Who has most credibility? Consider a situation in which it is just a small study, requiring the work to be done by one person. If, for example, the social worker for a number of people living in a house wanted to know how happy the people were with their accommodation, in order to plan further schemes, would he or she really be the best person to ask them? Would they be most open with the social worker or perhaps just tell him or her what they thought ought to be said. If someone recognized difficulties in a community house staffed by nurses, would that person be the most appropriate person to evaluate the situation if he or she were not a nurse? Or would that person be seen as interfering?

As mentioned previously, how to feed back the information? If parents/clients are asking for a study, they might be interested in a different type of presentation and feedback of information to a Ph.D. student doing a study for his or her own personal qualification. It may be that parents/clients are interested in descriptive accounts or videos, especially if they want to use these to illustrate the service to other interested families. A Ph.D. student may be much more concerned that he or she has some impressive statistics, lots of references, and 20,000 words! If a management committee is asking for the evaluation in order to consider the establishment of further community projects, they too could find a Ph.D. thesis difficult to wade through.

Consider also, and build into the study, how the information will be used. Some ideas will be described later in the illustrative study.

This chapter will now describe a study in which the author has been involved, following through the process described so far. This study is an evaluation of small staffed homes for children and young people who have recently moved out of local hospitals. There are four houses, each for six young people. At the time of writing the project was at the pilot stage. The intention is to undertake a 5-year study with annual collection of information.

So the first question: what is the study for, what point is to be proven? Explicitly the study is examining whether the service is doing what it says it is doing. There is an operational policy available. Why was the study started? Service evaluation was built into the operational policy and the original intention has been that evaluation would take place at the time the houses were opening. However, essentially this was a new local service and not a research programme, and so everyone was carried along with the natural enthusiasm of a new service. If there was a choice between service needs and research needs, then of course service needs came first. Those eventually involved in the study were very involved in the setting up and supporting of the new service that they did not want to see it failing. There may not, in fact, have been the same degree of interest and support in research evaluation then as there hopefully was later.

The request for evaluation eventually came through the Unit Management Team in the District Health Authority. Their interest, and subsequently the involvement of the Health and Social Services Joint Management Group, was to gain information for further planning of mental handicap services. How did the process occur? It was not very clear initially exactly what was wanted (apart from how much it would cost!) and so very detailed proposals were drawn up of what was to be collected, who would be involved in collecting it, how frequently the information would be collected, how much time it would take, what sort of computer would be needed, how much time would be involved in inputting, analysis, and reporting, and even how many photocopies would be needed! Hopefully, nobody was going to complain afterwards that they had not been told something!

The involvement of others was a very important aspect. In particular those considered as 'stakeholders' – that is, those who had something to gain, or feared they had something to lose. The Nurse Manager of all the houses was involved from the very start. He added information to the data collection which was of particular interest to him on various staff measures – for example, staff sickness, staff satisfaction, and reasons for leaving. This increased his commitment to the study and his support and encouragement of his staff to work with the study.

Part of the study involved gaining information on changes in the young people's behaviour outside of the homes, i.e. at school. In order to gain commitment to the study from education, an educational psychologist was invited to become a member of the team which developed the original proposals, thereby making him a dedicated 'stakeholder'.

Some of the information was to be made available to parents of the young people, and so they were involved by asking them to make comments on the suggestions for the pilot study, and designing the parental satisfaction questionnaire. No parents were on the group which developed the pilot project. The proposals may have been quite different if a representative parent had been involved. The slant of the project would probably have been slightly more towards asking whether the service was doing what parents wanted it to do. Following the pilot project, it is likely that a parent will be invited to join the group making proposals for the full evaluation.

How will the report back be managed? The results are for two groups, the Management Group and the parents. Most of the data will be presented to the Management Group in the form of an annual report. This might not be interesting or relevant for families, who might be more interested in exactly how the young people and the houses look, so videos will be used in the form of 'a day in the life of'. On the one hand, therefore, there will be descriptive accounts of changes in the young people in the houses over the 5 years of the study, and on the other hand visual images on video. How will results be utilized? It is expected that some recommendations will come out of the study. From the staff's point of view, for example, the most efficient ways of collecting information; from the manager's point of view, information on staff satisfaction and ideas on how to improve this; from the young people's point of view, more information on the effectiveness of the review system; and from the family's point of view, feedback to the staff on how they view the functioning of the home, support for staff, and ideas for change.

It is hoped that there will be a feedback loop through the houses, so that the study will have some sort of dynamic process, whereby results will be fed back to staff and families, used, possibly new ideas generated, which in turn are fed back into the study next time round. If, for example, parents became particularly interested in the study and asked for different sorts of information to be collected, these could be incorporated.

Similarly, if certain information, for example the videoing, were found to be intrusive, that could be reduced, If certain house procedures were found to be particularly stressful or dissatisfying for staff, then perhaps these could be altered and the changes in staff procedures subsequently measured. Part of the purpose of the pilot stage was to give more information on the most appropriate methods of feedback. One way of describing the study is as an 'action-research' model.

This is a summary of all the measures which are being collected (further information is available on request): client skills, client health status, use of general and mental handicap services, contact with family and friends and family satisfaction, goal achievement through the review system, staff measures, neighbourhood relations, client behaviour outside the home, general appearance of the clients and house through using video, and assessment of adherence to house philosophy through a PASS evaluation.

So what action in particular is it hoped will follow from the study? It should act as an external monitoring procedure to ensure that goals and plans are regularly made and followed through for the young people in the houses; there will be a closer examination of physical and social integration than might normally be achieved through individual's reviews; information will be collected on what families feel about the houses and whether any changes can be made if appropriate; staff satisfaction and difficulties should be identified and difficulties acted upon if necessary; a PASS evaluation will take place in order to advise on improvements in the quality of the service; and, hopefully, the Management Group will use the information to plan further housing in future, perhaps even smaller housing. The study is specifically looking at service change, and not individual or community change. It may also be that the evaluation will become a creative way of buying videos for the houses!

ACKNOWLEDGEMENTS

I wish to acknowledge the immense time and support given by Morag Hunter during the preparation of this chapter, and discussion with Morag, Ellie Stirling, and Sue Stirling which crystallized many of the ideas presented here.

REFERENCES

Felce, D., de Kock, U., Saxby, H., and Thomas, M. (1985) *Small Homes for Severely and Profoundly Mentally Handicapped Adults*, University of Southampton: Health Care Evaluation Research Team.

Heal, L. W. and Chadsey-Rusch, J. (1985) 'The Lifestyle Satisfaction Scale (LSS): assessing individual's satisfaction with residence, community setting and associated services', *Applied Research in Mental Retardation* 6 (4): 475–90.

King's Fund (1980) *'An Ordinary Life'. Comprehensive Locally-based Residential Services for Mentally Handicapped People*, King's Fund Centre, 126 Albert Street, London.

——(1983) *A Checklist of Twenty Questions: Creating Local Psychiatric Services*, London: King's Fund Centre.
——(1986) *Living Well into Old Age. Applying Principles of Good Practice to Services for People with Dementia*, London: King's Fund Centre.
MIND (1983) *Common Concern: MIND's Manifesto for a Comprehensive Mental Health Service*, 22 Harley Street, London WIN 2ED.
Newcastle Health Authority (undated) 'Small staffed homes. Operational policy', available from the Senior Assistant Director of Nursing, Mental Handicap Community Nursing, Newcastle upon Tyne.
Northumberland Area Health Authority (1981) '224 Alexandra Road Ashington – Operational Policy', available from The Director of Nursing Services, Northumberland, Health Authority, Morpeth.
Passfield, D. (1983) 'What do you think of it so far? A survey of 20 Priory Court residents', *Mental Handicap* 11 (3): 97–9.
Williams, A. (1986) 'The use of costs and outcome measures in establishing priorities in health care', paper presented at the NHSTA/DPS Management Course of District Clinical Psychologists, Harrogate.

Chapter Thirteen

NEED IN THE COMMUNITY

A district model[1]

GEOFF SHEPHERD

Fulbourn Hospital is situated about 4 miles from the centre of the city of Cambridge. A large, private housing estate has recently been completed next to the hospital, thus joining it to the suburbs. Cambridge is roughly in the middle of the Cambridge Health Authority catchment area, which has a current population of around 260,000. For many years Fulbourn was the only psychiatric facility in this area and the effective catchment area was therefore rather larger (?350,000). It is the region's policy that all districts should become self-sufficient in psychiatric services by the end of this strategic planning cycle (1994).

In total, we estimate that there are between 400 and 450 people living in the Health District who require some sort of asylum[2] due to the effects of long-term mental illness. Most of these are in contact with the Cambridge Psychiatric Rehabilitation Service (CPRS) which is based in the hospital. They can be divided into two groups: those currently living in the community, and those currently living on the hospital site. Those currently living in the community are a mixture of people who have been discharged from the hospital as part of a gradual process of reduction in numbers of long-stay patients which has been going on for almost 20 years, and 'new' long-term patients who have accumulated in the mean time and who have been maintained in the community, thereby being prevented from becoming new long-stay in-patients.

The process of resettlement of long-stay patients began in the 1950s and since then the hospital has reduced in size from more than 1,000 beds overall to less than 450 today.

There are currently around 120 places available in a range of sheltered accommodation in the community. These include:

(a) forty-five places in three staffed hostels – two run by a housing association and one by a voluntary body. These units provide 24-hour supervision and individual treatment and skills training. There are close links between these facilities and CPRS staff.

(b) thirty places in eight supported group homes – one run by Social Services and the others by a housing association. These are small units, generally two to three people, in ordinary houses. Care staff visit every weekday up to 20 hours per week and provide help and supervision with daily living-skills. Hospital staff (mainly CPNs) provide clinical support and for the housing association homes there is a joint management committee.

(c) forty-five places in twelve unstaffed group homes – four of these are hospital group homes and the other are run by voluntary agencies (including the local Mental Welfare Association). These homes are not staffed, but they are regularly visited.

Most of the hostel places are designed to be transitional and fairly short-term (up to 2 years) whereas the group homes offer permanent residence. Although we are reasonably well provided with sheltered accommodation, we recognize a need for more permanent hostel places and a housing association is about to open a new long-term hostel for eight residents later this month. In addition to those living in sheltered accommodation, the CPRS – particularly its CPNs – also offer support and treatment to patients living in their own homes and to their families. Between forty and fifty people receive this kind of support.

All the patients who are living in the community have access to a range of day facilities. There are currently around 160 day places available in a number of different units. These include approximately 100 places, providing sheltered work – about a half of these are on the hospital site, the remainder being in the city in two workshops, one run by Social Services and the other by a voluntary agency. A wide variety of work is available, including traditional packing and assembly, furniture restoring, toy making, horticulture, printing, and repairing bicycles.

The hospital workshops include a small unit (twelve places) funded by the Manpower Services Commission which aims to assess and prepare people who have had a mental illness for return to open employment. This is an experimental venture and is in the second of 3 years of initial funding. We have also recently appointed a part-time supervisor to run a Sheltered Placements Scheme (SPS) for eight to ten psychiatrically disabled clients. This involves placing disabled people in open industry with appropriate support.

There are also approximately sixty day places providing other therapies and social support – twenty of which are on the hospital site, the remainder being in the community in two units, one funded by the Health Authority and the other by a voluntary body.

We recognize the need to provide more day care away from the hospital site and there are plans to move one workshop (twenty-five places) out of the hospital and to set up a new day centre (between twenty-five and thirty places) for the long-term mentally ill as part of a joint project with Social Services. This will be run along similar lines to 'Fountain House' (Beard et al. 1982) and should be operational within the next two years.

Turning now to the long-stay patients in hospital, the vast majority are elderly (two-thirds are over 65) and most have spent many years in hospital (mean length of stay 21 years). About one-quarter have moderate to severe physical disabilities.

Their needs are illustrated in Table 13.1, which shows the results of a dependency survey carried out using the Clifton Assessment Procedure for the Elderly (CAPE). This suggests that three-quarters show levels of dependency equal to or greater than people living in residential homes for the elderly. Given the shortage of permanent hostel provision mentioned earlier, it is

Table 13.1 CAPE scores for long-stay patients at Fulbourn Hospital (1983)

N = 130 *Mean age: 63 years (range 30–85)* *Mean length of admission: 21 yrs (range 1–54 yrs)*	*N*	%
(A) No impairment: independent elderly	11	8
(B) Mild impairment: low dependency	22	17
(C) Moderate impairment: medium dependency	44	35
(D) Marked impairment: high dependency	37	28
(E) Severe impairment: maximum dependency	16	12

difficult to see how they might be offered a better quality of care outside the hospital. It is therefore the Health Authority's intention to reprovide suitable accommodation for these patients on the hospital site.

In the mean time, we have been attempting to move as many patients as possible out of the Victorian wards of the institution and into ordinary houses in the hospital grounds. Some of these projects use existing nursing staff as the primary carers; in other cases we have again worked with a local housing association and used the residents' DHSS benefits to employ care assistants. All these projects have ready access to the facilities already available at the hospital, particularly the day services.

At present we have about twenty patients living in such accommodation and we have plans to develop another two or three houses offering an additional 20–25 places. We have also just opened a 'hospital hostel' (ward-in-a-house) in the grounds for new long-stay in-patients. This will offer long-term, intensive rehabilitation in a domestic setting for a small group of initially eight residents, all of whom have spent at least a year continuously in hospital. It is modelled on units already in existence at the Maudsley, Southampton, and Manchester.

For the future, we estimate a need of about 120 long-stay beds in 1994. This is based on statistical projections carried out by Dr Tim Moore of the Department of Community Medicine using data collected by myself and another psychologist, Barbie Antonis (Moore et al. 1987). This data consisted of a follow-up of 153 patients admitted to the rehabilitation service between 1970 and 1980. The outcome of each patient was determined and a mathematical model constructed describing the relationship between length of stay and probability of discharge (as length of stay increases so probability of discharge decreases). Then, using the age profile of the existing long-stay patients and their age-specific mortality rates, it is possible to predict the rate of decline of this population over the 10-year period. This is shown in the middle line of Figure 13.1

In order to estimate the total need for long-stay places, we must add to this the number of 'new' long-stay in-patients likely to accumulate. Once again this is obtained by taking local data on the numbers of new referrals over the past few years and then applying the model. Our annual incidence rates for potential new long-stay

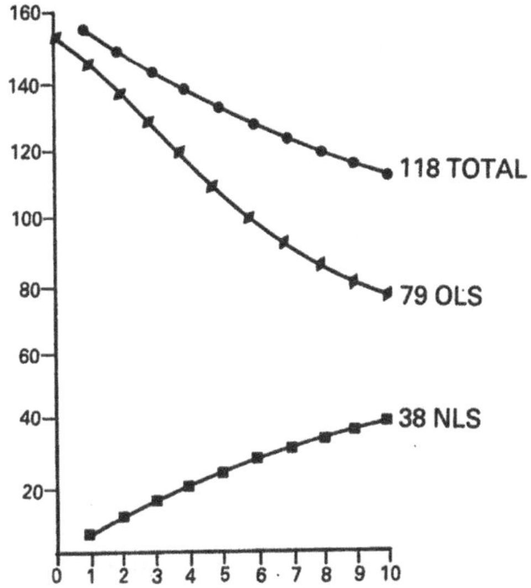

Figure 13.1 Projected bed needs for Cambridge Health Authority (Pop. 262,000) for existing (old) long-stay, new long-stay, and total

in-patients (6–8 per year) are similar to the median rates from other case registers (around 3–4 per 100,000) reported by Gibbons et al. (1984). These comparative data also show marked regional variation, underlining the need for local models. Our figures predict a rate of accumulation which is shown in the bottom line of Figure 13.1.

Adding these two curves together gives the estimated total need and this is shown in the upper line. The figures given here represent the mid range and they are consistent with the projections based on national, DHSS data (Robertson 1981). He suggests that, 'unless there is a radical departure from current practice', the number of beds likely to be occupied in 1991 for lengths of stay of more than one year amount to 53 per 100,000 (including those over 65, but excluding dementias).

It should be emphasized here that, technically, these data apply to *people* and not to beds. Thus, they suggest that there may be 120 people requiring the kind of service we normally associate with long stay beds. They do not preclude the possibility that this need may be met with a different kind of service.

In general then, we have chosen to retain a fairly substantial proportion of our asylum provision on the hospital site – at least in the medium-term future. We would argue that this is justifiable given the needs of these patients in terms of day activities, medical and nursing care, and the relatively good accessibility of the hospital to the community. Purchasing alternative property or land would be very expensive and we believe that it is better to use the existing site and to sell parts of it to finance redevelopment, rather than to plan for a totally devolved service. The site will also continue to be used by other parts of the mental health service and, with the advent of a direct bus route through the grounds, we think that it should be possible to maintain an open, community-oriented institution.

We thus agree with the House of Commons Social Services Committee (1985) where they recommend:

> that no mental illness or mental handicap hospital site be disposed of without explicit consideration being given to the possible redevelopment of suitable parts for mental disability services and that redevelopment should have to be justifiable solely on the intrinsic merits of the proposals, and not rely simply on the availability of the land (para. 208).

The interface between the hospital and the community is well reflected in the work of the CPRS intake ward. This unit, which is currently located on the hospital site, acts mainly as an acute admission ward for long-term patients from the community who are suffering acute relapses. It also screens potential new long-stay in-patients and refers them on to the hospital hostel where appropriate. As the services in the community have developed, particularly the range of sheltered housing, it has become increasingly clear that the follow-up and support of these 'revolving door' patients has not been adequate.

The next major development for the rehabilitation service is therefore to move this unit into the community and to increase its staffing so as to be able to provide much more flexible support for people wherever they are living. It is hoped that a flexible and mobile 'community team', with the back-up of a residential unit for short admissions, will help maintain patients for longer periods without recourse to hospital and will provide much-needed support for residential staff, many of whom are quite inexperienced in the care of the long-term mentally ill. It may also be a way of beginning to monitor quality and standards of care in what has rapidly become a multi-site and multi-agency service.

To summarize, then, we believe that there is a substantial need for 'asylum' but that it can take many forms. Peoples' needs for shelter and support vary both across time and across different areas of their lives. Services therefore need to be organized so as to be able to meet these needs in the most flexible and economic way.

Most of these solutions consist of various kinds of partial asylum with combinations of sheltered accommodation and sheltered daytime activities.

'Asylum' can therefore be a positive, as well as a negative, concept. A good quality of care may be provided in a segregated setting, although generally it is more difficult. On the other hand, care in the community is not, by itself, a guarantee that either good quality care, or an enhanced quality of life will necessarily occur. Quality and location of care must therefore be clearly separated (Shepherd 1984).

Patients have a right to be with other patients sometimes, just as they have a right to be with so-called 'normal' people. The problem is how to give them these opportunities without either imprisoning them in the sick role, or denying their disabilities. Trying to pretend that either does not exist is really just to close one's eyes to the reality of the problem.

NOTES

1. This chapter was originally presented as a paper at a consensus development conference on 'The need for asylum in society for the mentally ill or infirm', King's Fund Centre, 8–10 April 1987. It is reproduced by permission of the King's Fund Centre.
2. This refers to any kind of specialized service (in-patient admission, day care, out-patient, or domiciliary care) required because of the disabling effects of long-term mental illness.

REFERENCES

Beard, J. H., Propst, R. N., and Malamud, T. J. (1982) 'The Fountain House model of psychiatric rehabilitation', *Psychosocial Rehabilitation*

Journal 5: 47–59.
Gibbons, J., Jennings, C., and Wing, J. K. (1984) *Psychiatric care in eight register areas*', Knowle Hospital, Southampton: Southampton Psychiatric Case Register.
House of Commons (1985) *Second Report from the Social Services Committee on Community Care*, London: HMSO.
Moore, T. J., Shepherd, G., and Antonis, B. (1987) Long stay psychiatric bed requirements: A planning model. Paper in preparation, Department of Community Medicine, Cambridge Health Authority.
Robertson, G. (1981) 'Provision of in-patient facilities for the mentally ill: a paper to assist NHS planners', London: DHSS.
Shepherd, G. (1984) *Institutional Care and Rehabilitation*, London: Longmans

Chapter Fourteen

QUALITY IN RESIDENTIAL SERVICES FOR ADULTS WITH SEVERE OR PROFOUND MENTAL HANDICAP

Lessons from a development project

DAVID FELCE

A major change in social policy has been initiated in the last two decades concerned with the replacement of institutional provision by services on a more human scale. Institutional care has been criticized for its inhumane or extremely poor treatment of its charges (Blatt and Kaplan 1966; DHSS 1969; Morris 1969; Oswin 1971). Researchers writing on the origins, purposes, and working regimes of institutions have demonstrated the lack of relationship between institutional characteristics and the welfare of their inmates (Goffman 1961; Wolfensberger 1969). Policies of reform have strengthened, and these have derived momentum from the deinstitutionalization movement, the elaboration of the principle of normalization (Wolfensberger 1972; Wolfensberger and Glenn 1975), statements concerning the rights of individuals to live in the community and to live in the least restrictive environment possible, and a complementary recognition of the abilities and potential of people with mental handicap (O'Connor and Tizard 1951, 1956; Clarke and Hermelin 1955; Berkson and Landesman-Dwyer 1977).

It is important to recognize that these changes have been relatively recent. So too have our attempts to provide alternative services (for example Tizard 1964; Kushlick 1970; Mathieson and Blunden 1980; Mansell et al. 1983; Ward 1983) or to conduct research which addresses the quality of different types of residential experience. In developing a scale to encapsulate the quality of residential care as 'client-orientated', or 'administration-orientated', King et al. (1971) made the first significant attempt in this country to quantify the quality of day-to-day existence for people with mental handicap in residential services as distinct from more traditional measures of treatment outcome.

The evaluation of the first community-based alternatives to institutional care in Wessex incorporated a variety of measurement approaches to represent the impact of the services on their users (Felce, Kushlick, and Smith 1980). By the very fact of the extent of time that people depend on them, residential services exert a major influence over their users' lives. Moreover, home life has many facets. Residential services must therefore seek to promote positive outcomes for the people served on a number of dimensions of personal welfare. I have argued elsewhere that the evaluation of quality is best achieved by adopting a range of measurement approaches which match the range of functions and accomplishments appropriate to a housing service (Felce 1986; 1987a). This viewpoint has also underpinned the evaluation approach being taken in relation to the NIMROD service (Humphreys et al. 1986) and is consistent with the view of O'Brien (1987) that there are a number of distinct accomplishments which a high-quality human service should strive to provide for its users.

This chapter has two purposes. Its first is to summarize in one place the major results of the evaluation of a housing service for adults with severe or profound mental handicaps (and some with challenging behaviour) which was set up in Winchester Health District (Mansell et al. 1983; Felce et al. 1984) as a second stage of community developments within Wessex. By this time one had not only been able to achieve a reduction in size of unit and the use of ordinary housing, but also (a) a very clear and specific statement of the objectives which the service would seek to achieve, and (b) the development of a number of related systematic approaches to guide how staff worked with and on behalf of residents.

The second purpose of this chapter is to set out the lessons learnt from that research. Why was it that the housing service was considerably better than the other facilities to which it was compared?

THE HOUSING MODEL

More complete descriptions of the way the houses were established and operated have already been given (Mansell et al. 1983; Felce et al. 1984; Mansell et al. 1987; Felce, 1987b). We were interested in developing a residential environment which gave the people living there effective opportunities to participate in a wide range of activity and to continue to grow in competence and experience. These objectives were set within a broader context of a continuing relationship with immediate family and an ordinary community life. To these ends, the residences were small, enriched, well staffed, managerially autonomous, and served people with local ties. They had a structured approach to individual plan review, to how staff arranged their responsibilities for resident care and the provision of activity, and to how staff supported residents in the conduct of the household routine. Considerable emphasis was also given to monitoring resident experience.

The first two houses were the subject of research. They provided eight places each and were both ordinary detached houses in residential neighbourhoods. They are situated a few minutes walk either side of the shopping centre of the main town in the catchment territory served. Each was equipped to a high material standard with an emphasis on retaining a fully domestic character. Environmental deprivation (for example, not having carpeting or breakable objects) or over-protection (for example vinyl-covered furniture) as resident management strategies were avoided and there was no restriction of resident access to areas which may be considered to have greater inherent risks such as the kitchen.

Each house had a person-in-charge, deputy, seven other day staff, and four half-time night staff. The day staff worked from 7.30 a.m. to 3.00 p.m. and from 2.30 p.m. to 10.00 p.m. with two or three staff on duty at a time. The care-staff role was to help residents lead as full an ordinary home life as possible, doing their own cooking and other domestic tasks. To support this orientation, the houses had considerable autonomy over budgeting and purchasing. They did not receive externally organized services such as centralized laundry or supply of provisions. Senior staff were responsible for house maintenance and recruitment of their junior staff.

The aim, which was to provide for each person the same range of home and community activities that are important to anyone else of similar age, was ambitious taking the level of handicap of the residents into account: all of the adults with the greatest handicaps who required residential care from the catchment area were served without exception. The service is a specialist one and the expression of that specialism is in the structured approach taken to staff performance and staff:resident interaction. Specific procedures promoted a goal-setting approach in the formulation of individual resident plans (Jenkins et al. in press), the writing of formal teaching programmes (Mansell et al. 1986), and daily plans by which staff decide how they are to involve all residents in activity during the day (Felce and de Kock, 1983; Brown and Brown, 1987; Mansell et al. 1987). Staff were taught to use an instruct/show/prompt/guide hierarchy to enable the residents to participate effectively but at the same time as independently as possible. Staff were also taught to motivate resident participation by giving attention contingent on engagement in activity. During the course of each day, staff recorded what household and community activities residents had been involved in, the implementation and success of teaching, and any social contact residents had with family or friends. This information was summarized to provide a source of feedback and critical review at the two- to three-hour weekly staff meeting.

THE EVALUATION OF RESIDENT EXPERIENCE: AN OVERVIEW OF RESULTS

The evaluation was concerned to assess the extent to which the housing service achieved its aims to promote (a) active participation in daily living, household, and community activities; (b) skill development over time; and (c) involvement in the community and social life of the local town. Measures were therefore defined in these areas and the experiences of the residents of the housing project compared with those in hospital settings and in larger community-based units, similar to those which we had evaluated in our previous research in Wessex. The research used between-group and within-group comparative designs.

The residents of the houses were demonstrated in the course of the research to be representative of the most handicapped adults in residential care. The group included people who had been characterized as severely behaviour disordered for many years and who had been living in specially restricted institutional environments immediately prior to transfer to the houses.

Engagement in activity: studies of participation within the houses

Study One (Mansell, Jenkins, Felce and de Kock 1984)

Residents of the first house observed over five week days between 7.00 to 10.00 a.m. and 3.00 to 11.00 p.m. spent

- an average of 46% of their time actively participating in a range of personal, domestic, leisure and social activity;
- between 27% and 65% of that time involved in domestic activity with domestic activity comprising over half of the active engagement of four of the six residents.

Studies Two and Three (Felce, de Kock, and Repp, 1986; Felce, Thomas, de Kock, Saxby, and Repp, 1985)

Engagement levels during several three-hour periods centred on the evening meal per person were contrasted in a three-way comparison involving (a) residents of the first house, (b) the future residents of the second house while they were still living in hospital settings, and (c) the residents of the second house about three months after they had moved into the housing scheme.
House residents spent:

- 51% and 56% of their time actively participating in a range of personal, domestic, and leisure pursuits compared with a pre-transfer level of 23% while in hospital;
- 17% and 14% of their time in social interaction compared with only 1% in hospital;
- nearly twice as much time actively manipulating materials and utensils in their environment than when in hospital in over twice as many categories of activities.

Study Four (Thomas, Felce, de Kock, Saxby, and Repp, 1986)

Five matched groups of ten residents in two hospitals, two large community units, and the small homes respectively were each observed between 8.30 a.m. and 6.00 p.m. (omitting meal times) on two days.
House residents spent:

- 40% of their time adaptively engaged in personal, domestic, and leisure pursuits compared with 11% for residents in the large community units and 3% for residents in hospital;

- 7% of their time in social interaction with staff compared with 1% in both the large community units and hospitals; and
- 6% of their time in inappropriate activity compared with 13% for residents in the large community units and 27% for those in hospitals.

Engagement in activity: studies of participation in community amenities

Study One (de Kock et al. 1988)

The frequency of going to (a) shops (b) pubs, restaurants, and cafés, (c) cultural or leisure events, or (d) some other excursion into the community was recorded for residents of the houses, and compared with the level of community use experienced in their prior institutional settings and to that of similar residents in large community units.
House residents had an average of:

- 254 community excursions per year (range, 126–424) compared with 71 (range, 0–178) for residents of the large community units and seven (range, 0–52) when in hospitals.
- 140 trips shopping each per year and forty-eight opportunities each to go out to eat or drink.

Study Two (Saxby et al. 1986)

Ten residents of the houses were observed on a number of occasions each while shopping or going to a pub, café, or restaurant to assess their level of participation in activity appropriate to the setting.
House residents spent:

- 29% and 36% of their time in shops and in pubs, cafés, or restaurants respectively participating in activity appropriate to the setting;
- 6% and 11% respectively engaged in social interaction with members of the household party;
- 2% and 2% engaged in social interaction with members of the public; and
- 6% and 11% respectively engaged in inappropriate activity.

Developmental progress (Felce, de Kock, Thomas, and Saxby 1986)

The progress of the residents of the houses was compared against similar individuals living in long-stay hospitals or their family homes using the AAMD Adaptive Behavior Scale Part One (Nihira et al. 1974), the Griffiths Mental Development Scales (Griffiths 1954, 1971) and the Reynell Developmental Language Scales (Reynell 1977).
House residents:

- progressed more than institutional residents or adults living with their families;
- made greatest progress in the areas of independent functioning, domestic activity, and self-direction (as defined in the Adaptive Behavior Scale);
- made progress irrespective of initial extent of disability or other impairments.

Family and friendship contact (de Kock et al. 1988)

The frequencies of being visited by and going out for the day or overnight stays with family or friends (not staff or volunteers) were recorded for residents of the houses, and compared with the levels of such events experienced in their prior institutional settings and by similar residents in large community units.
House residents had an average of:

- 74 family and friendship contacts per year (range, 10–182) compared to 48 (range, 0–140) for residents of the large community units and 11 (range, 0–36) when in hospitals.

EXPLAINING THE DIFFERENCES IN RESULTS

The evaluation shows that in many areas of daily living, range of environmental opportunity and appropriate stimulation the housing service was greatly superior. The important question to address is 'Why'? – for if it is possible to answer this question, then we will know what it is important to attend to when attempting to bring about similar improvements in the course of providing alternative services for the many thousands of people who live in inferior residential settings. A major programme of reform is beginning: it is vital that the new services being developed are based on an understanding of how best to benefit the service user.

It is quite clear that the lessons are not simple ones. It is common sense that the houses were not of high quality simply because they were small and architecturally ordinary. Research has shown that factors such as size of residence or staffing level, which are at the very heart of major policy arguments, have little effect on quality *in themselves* (i.e. on their own) (for example, Balla 1976; Landesman-Dwyer, Sackett and Kleinman 1980; Landesman-Dwyer 1981). It is quite easy to conceive of a badly run, isolated housing scheme providing an unstimulating 'hotel' service, cut off from the surrounding community and in which the very handicapped residents living there have few opportunities and do little during the day.

In the remainder of this chapter, I have tried to address this essential question by drawing on other research studies which we conducted as part of the overall evaluation as well as the wider behavioural literature. I will deal first with three sets of factors which are related to the extent to which residents engage in appropriate daily living activities.

Factors related to engagement

The supportive model

The literature in general (for example, Warren and Mondy, 1971; Wright et al. 1974; Moores and Grant, 1976; Repp and Barton, 1980) has shown very low rates of interaction between staff and severely or profoundly mentally handicapped residents. The pattern of staff–resident interaction in these houses was markedly different. Interactions occurred at a high rate and the extent of support given was related to resident ability. Felce, de Kock, and Repp (1986) showed residents in the houses received instruction from staff for 19.8% and 11.3% of their time, on average, and physical guidance for 5.2% and 3.2%. Comparable levels in hospitals were 1.0% and zero. Levels of staff support were shown to vary inversely with the residents' mental ages, with the most handicapped getting more staff support. Finally, the association between staff instruction and guidance on the one hand and resident engagement on the other was shown by a Spearman rank

Staff – resident interactions

◊ Instruct

◊ Show

◊ Prompt

◊ Guide

THE SUPPORTIVE MODEL

implies need:

* material enrichment
* task-analytic skill
* an orientation to produce staff support rather than staff doing things to or for residents
* to avoid separate domestic and catering staff and the use of works department, or other central services, e.g. linen and laundry

Figure 14.1 The supportive model

correlation coefficient of 0.97, calculated on within-subject differences across pairs of data.

Our research showed that staff were implementing their training on how to support the participation of very handicapped people by extensive use of a hierarchy of antecedent conditions – instruct/show/prompt/guide (Figure 14.1). This aspect of staff performance is therefore a critical determinant of quality. However, other factors contribute to the staff's ability to work in this way.

Material enrichment is a logical precondition of any level of day-to-day activity. We all need many objects to pursue our varied home lives. It is particularly relevant in the case of residents who have considerable handicaps and largely lack language. Not only were materials important to much of the routine personal, household, and leisure activities followed, but they were also important in the transaction of social interaction.

The task-analytic skill which had actually been taught to staff for the purpose of structuring skill-teaching was also relevant to the way they began to conduct daily life. Staff became adept at conceiving of complex domestic tasks as chains of simple behaviours. Each step could be prompted or assisted in turn. Thus, no task was beyond the capability of the most handicapped person to carry out with assistance.

Certain traditional practices had to be abandoned in order for this orientation to be pursued to the full. Staff had to adopt a role of supporting residents to do things for themselves rather than staff doing them on their behalf. Staff had to resist getting the chores done quickly in order to create time to spend with the clients. Rather, they spent all of their time with the residents helping them to get the chores done. Decisions had been taken in the planning of these houses that there would be no domestic or catering staff (using the revenue allocations that would have been used to establish more care-staff posts). This had been done to allow residents access to a full range of activity. One could not expect to employ domestic staff and cooks without them doing the cleaning and cooking and, thereby, denying these opportunities to residents. Similarly, other forms of 'hotel' service such as centralized laundry and works department cover were rejected; available revenue being channelled into the budget devolved to the staff running the houses.

The motivational model

Not only has the frequency of staff interaction with mentally handicapped residents been traditionally low, it has not always encouraged appropriate participation when it has occurred (for example, Thormahlen, 1965; Warren and Mondy, 1971; Whatmore et al. 1975; Repp and Barton 1983). The 'room management' projects demonstrated how changing the distribution of staff attention (towards attending to people when engaged appropriately) could benefit activity patterns (for example, Porterfield et al. 1980; McBrien and Weightman 1980; Mansell et al. 1982). Following the general principle rather than the specific application demonstrated by this research staff in the houses had therefore been taught to give their attention to residents when they were involved in household or other daily living activity (Figure 14.2).

A study of institutions, large community units, and small houses that we conducted to shed light on this aspect of the residential

Staff – resident interactions:

◊ the frequency and

◊ contingency

of

◊ attention and praise

THE MOTIVATIONAL MODEL

implies need:

* the supportive model to create engagement for people with severe or profound handicaps

Figure 14.2 The motivational model

setting (Felce et al. 1987) showed that staff attention was directed more to appropriate participation in the houses than in other settings. Over three-quarters of staff attention was given to residents when they were engaged in appropriate activity and almost three-fifths of appropriate resident behaviour was contacted by staff within the 15-second interval in which it occurred.

For very handicapped people, the motivational model is hard to implement without the supportive model (see, for example, the demonstration of a 'low-engagers' group and the discussion of that finding in the 'room-management' study by Mansell et al. 1982). The supportive model is required to create the initial adaptive participation which can then be the focus of staff attention in order to bring the motivational model into play. Individuals who, when first admitted to the houses, had little inclination to initiate or persist in meaningful activities have learnt to do so through many months and years of exposure to this kind of motivational climate (see Felce and Toogood 1988).

Working conditions:

◊ size of staff – resident group

◊ planned activities and staff deployment

◊ monitoring and feedback

THE ORGANIZATIONAL MODEL

implies need:

* small size
* domestic design
* to plan meeting and review time into staff rotas
* systems for organization and recording

Figure 14.3 The organizational model

The organizational model

More attention and debate has been given to the issue of size of residence than just about any other factor in the design of residential provision. Yet little is known about the direct effects which facility size exerts on the life-style of residents. A complementary study on the houses, hospitals, and large community units (Felce et al. in press) looked at the relationship between the size of staff and resident group and staff and resident behaviour. We looked at resident engagement and staff–resident interactions in the same way as in the other studies described above, but also recorded the number of residents and number of staff in the room occupied by the person being observed. We were then able to analyse activity patterns by size of resident group: 1, 2–4, 5–9, 10 or more (in the large settings) or 1, 2, 3 (in the houses) each according to whether one, two, or three staff were present.

The desirable situations were when staff worked on their own with 1–4 residents. When the resident group was 5–9 or 10 or more, staff interactions and resident engagement were low irrespective of whether there were one, two, or three staff present. Even when the resident group was small, it did not improve matters for two or three staff to be present; often it meant that less was achieved than when one member of staff worked alone. Planning staff deployment so that staff have separate responsibilities for the care of individuals is a desirable practice (Figure 14.3).

A system of daily planning was followed in the houses so that staff–resident groupings were not left to chance (Felce and de Kock 1983). The prime function was for staff to determine their own deployment to work with residents so that all residents had a single identified staff member responsible for them at all times. Each staff member's job was to create opportunities for their residents to engage in activity within the context of a weekly household routine.

A second function of the planning system was to provide a method of keeping track of the opportunities each resident was given to engage in activity. Several studies in the applied research literature indicate that some form of monitoring and feedback is necessary in the establishment and maintenance of desirable staff behaviour. One should not overlook the role of organization and structure in the explanation of quality.

The organizational model also suggests the desirability of certain underlying structures to the provision of residential services. The size and design of ordinary housing may more naturally produce the staff–resident groupings found to be desirable. The smaller initial resident group and therefore staff establishment limits the extent to which a system of planning and communication is needed to subdivide the total group to create the working conditions associated with desirable practice. The variety of domestic-scale activity areas each of different function found in ordinary housing also strongly promotes separation into one-to-one or one-to-small-group working. Finally, it is important to design the staff rota to allow full, weekly staff meetings to take account of the information monitored.

Factors related to development

Developmental progress as a goal of services for people with mental handicap has assumed central importance in recent years. To this end, emphasis has been put on the need for individual, structured programmes which develop new and change existing patterns of behaviour. However there has been a tendency to divorce or at least fail to relate individual programming to what happens at other times of the person's day. Figure 14.4 sets out what I have termed 'The whole of life model'. This sets specific programming for both teaching new skills and developing alternatives to challenging behaviours within a more general environmental context. The development found in the small homes is seen not only as a consequence of individual teaching or behavioural intervention but also of the widespread opportunities to use skills and learn from routine experience which a high level of engagement and contingent staff interaction provide.

Staff of the houses had two mechanisms for targeting individual skill development: structured individual teaching programmes (Mansell et al. 1986) and less structured goal-planning (Toogood et al. 1983). They also formulated individual strategies to reduce difficult behaviours and replace them with more constructive behaviours. However, although these kinds of programmes and the programming skills of staff are absolutely necessary to the kind of success obtained, they may not be effective on their own. Certainly, effectiveness is enhanced in a setting in which routine engagement is the predominant feature. Skill acquisition and behaviour modification have to be part of everyday life, not a tacked-on marginal addition. The reasons for this are not simply philosophical but also practical.

It is common sense but also repeatedly referred to in the behavioural literature that (a) skills do not maintain if unused, and (b) long-term suppression of difficult behaviour cannot be achieved unless alternative behaviours are encouraged to take their place. One must therefore create a milieu which supports and encourages a wide range of adaptive and pro-social activity. In looking to explain the beneficial development of the small home residents, one would therefore not only point to the systems programming but also to those factors which are crucial to the supportive, motivational, and organizational models in the above analysis.

New skills

◊ Teaching programmes

◊ Learning from experience

◊ Opportunities to use skills (relevance)

THE WHOLE OF LIFE MODEL

implies need:

* high level and variety of engagement
* supportive and motivational models

Alternatives to challenging behaviour

◊ Intervention programmes

◊ Support alternative behaviours

◊ Motivate alternative behaviours

implies need:

* high level of engagement
* supportive and motivational models

Figure 14.4 The whole of life model

Factors related to community integration and family and friendship contact

Directly analogous factors operate in the determination of the improved levels of community activity and contact with family and friends experienced by the small-home residents. These are summarized in Figure 14.5. Location is an important variable with two separate dimensions: location close to community amenities and location *vis-à-vis* a local client group and local next-of-kin (catchment area) In the same way that material enrichment may be considered a pre-condition of engagement, community location and proximity to community amenities and family may be considered pre-conditions of community activity and family contact. Distance between family home and residential services has been a consistently implicated factor in research on rate of contact (Campbell, 1968; Burrows et al. 1968; Ballinger, 1970; Balla and Zigler, 1971; McKeown et al. 1971; Anderson et al. 1975; Felce, Lunt and Kushlick, 1980). Distance can be viewed as representing a cluster of obstacles to contact. Once removed, the frequency of

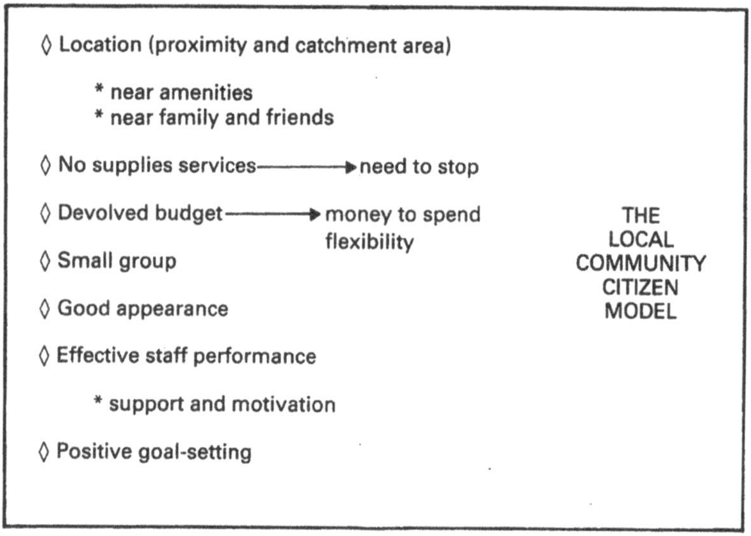

Figure 14.5 The local community citizen model

family and friendship contact may be open to influence by many other variables associated with the quality of the setting: from the many factors which have already been discussed which may promote activity and developmental progress to simple structural factors such as the availability of individual rooms to host visitors in reasonable comfort and privacy and access to those household resources required to offer normal hospitality.

In itself, physical location may not be considered a sufficient condition for high community use (for example, Birenbaum and Re, 1979). Certain other structural variables promote community integration: for example, the absence of centralized supply necessitates shopping and budget devolution, and gives staff flexibility to make many normal household decisions involving the use of community resources such as to eat out after shopping rather than to return for lunch. Although they were equally advantageously placed in terms of proximity to amenities, community use was less in the larger community units studied. One possible reason was that there was less need to use community resources and staff had less flexibility to do so because of a greater input of independently organized supply and catering services.

The level of participation when in community amenities of the house residents shows some evidence that staff generalized the approach taken to resident involvement within the homes to the world outside. The purpose of shopping was not seen simply as a means of obtaining provisions but also for promoting resident activity and experience. The level of integration was also found to be highly acceptable (Saxby et al. 1986). It is possible to characterize the good opinion of shopkeepers and bar staff as resting on an unstated bargain between the service and community. Groupings were normative: one or two residents with a member of staff while shopping and sometimes slightly larger parties for a social gathering in a pub. Considerable effort had been given to individuals having a good appearance appropriate to their chronological age. Staff were seen as diligent in their responsibility for resident behaviour. The residents were also clearly identifiable as financial contributors to the local economy. The lack of alternative means of procurement mentioned above resulted in residents shopping regularly (with staff) for a relatively large household. Full budget devolution has meant that, despite most being personally poor, residents have been able to act as ordinary consumers. Most businesses said they benefited from having them as customers. Two reasons were given: (a) the actual business done was worth having, and (b) a good public image was created by the business being open to handicapped members of the community.

CONCLUSION

The task of service providers is to arrange as many factors as possible to promote resident welfare. This and other research would suggest that it would be wrong to hope that high-quality outcome will be assured by correct determination of a few key variables in the structure of the service. My belief is that the entire range of factors discussed here contributes to resident experience. One would therefore urge service planners to be equally detailed in their task of determining the many working arrangements which constitute a residential environment. In doing so, one would also recommend the value of establishing coherence between the aims, structure, and procedures of the service. If planning decisions are to be based on rationales concerning consequences for residents, a prerequisite is an unambiguous statement of service aims: what the service seeks to accomplish for the user. This statement must then guide service structure and procedures so as to: (a) avoid creating obstacles to the achievement of resident objectives, (b) provide the conditions necessary for such achievement (i.e. opportunities), (c) create conditions favourable to staff to implement the staff performance desired, and (d) translate opportunity into achievement through attention to procedural systems designed to promote such desired staff performance.

REFERENCES

Anderson, W. H., Schlottman, R. S., and Weiner, B. J. (1975) 'Predictors of parent involvement with institutionalised retarded children', *American Journal of Mental Deficiency* 79: 705–10.

Balla, D. (1976) 'Relationship of institution size to quality care: a review of the literature', *American Journal of Mental Deficiency* 81: 117–24.

——and Zigler, E. (1971) 'The therapeutic role of visits and vacations for institutionalized retarded children', *Mental Retardation* 9: 7–9.

Ballinger, B. R. (1970) 'Community contacts of institutionalised mental

defectives', *British Journal of Mental Subnormality* 16: 17–23.
Berkson, G. and Landesman-Dwyer, S. (1977) 'Behavioural research on severe and profound mental retardation (1955–1974)', *American Journal of Mental Deficiency* 81: 428–54.
Birenbaum, A. and Re, M. A. (1979) 'Resettling mentally retarded adults in the community – almost 4 years later', *American Journal of Mental Deficiency* 83: 323–9.
Blatt, B. and Kaplan, F. (1966) *Christmas in Purgatory*, Boston: Allyn and Bacon.
Brown, V. and Brown, H. (1987) *Bringing People Back Home: Participation in Everyday Activities*, Brighton: ESCATA/SE Thames RHA.
Burrows, R. E., Pasewark, R. A., and Gillette, L. (1968) 'Visitation and vacation rates of the institutionally retarded', *Training School Bulletin* 65: 106–11.
Campbell, A. C. (1968) 'Comparison of family and community contacts of mentally subnormal adults in hospital and local authority hostels', *British Journal of Preventive Social Medicine* 22: 165–9.
Clarke, A. D. B. and Hermelin, B. F. (1955) 'Adult imbeciles: their abilities and trainability', *Lancet* ii: 337–9.
de Kock, U., Saxby, H. Thomas, M. and Felce, D., (1988) 'Community and family contact: an evaluation of small community homes for adults with severe and profound mental handicaps, *Mental Handicap Research* 1: 12–40.
Department of Health and Social Security (DHSS) (1969) *Report of the Committee of Inquiry into Allegations of Ill-treatment of Patients and Other Irregularities at the Ely Hospital, Cardiff*, Cmnd 3975, London: HMSO.
Felce, D. (1986) 'Housing for severely and profoundly mentally handicapped adults', in N. Eisenberg and D. Glasgow (eds) *Current Issues in Clinical Psychology: 1987 Annual Merseyside Course in Clinical Psychology*', Aldershot: Gower.
——(1987a) 'Evaluation by direct observation', in J. Beswick, T. Zadik, and D. Felce (eds) *Evaluating Quality of Care*, Kidderminster: BMIH Publications.
——(1987b) 'Behavioural and social climate in community residences', in M. Janicki, M. Krauss, and M. Seltzer (eds) *Here to Stay: Operating Community Residences*, Baltimore: Paul H. Brookes and Co.
——and de Kock, U. (1983) 'Planning client activity: a handbook', University of Southampton: Health Care Evaluation Research Team.
Felce, D. and Toogood, S. (1988) *Close to Home*, Kidderminster: BMIH Publications.
Felce, D., de Kock, U., and Repp, A. (1986) 'An eco-behavioural analysis of small community-based houses and traditional large hospitals for severely and profoundly mentally handicapped adults', *Applied Research in Mental Retardation* 7: 393–408.
Felce, D., Kushlick, A., and Smith, J. (1980) 'An overview of the research on alternative residential facilities for the severely mentally handicapped in Wessex', *Advances in Behavioural Research and Therapy* 3: 1–4.

Felce, D., Lunt, B., and Kushlick, A. (1980) 'Evaluation of alternative residential facilities for the severely mentally handicapped in Wessex: family contact', *Advances in Behaviour Research and Therapy* 3: 19–23.

Felce, D., de Kock, U., Saxby, H., and Thomas, M. (1985) 'Small homes for severely and profoundly mentally handicapped adults: final report', University of Southampton: Health Care Evaluation Research Team.

Felce, D., de Kock, U., Thomas, M., and Saxby, H. (1986) 'Change in adaptive behaviour of severely and profoundly mentally handicapped adults in different residential settings', *British Journal of Psychology* 77: 489–501.

Felce, D., Mansell, J., de Kock, U., Toogood, S., and Jenkins, J. (1984) 'Housing for severely and profoundly mentally handicapped adults', *Hospital and Health Service Review* 80: 170–4.

Felce, D., Thomas, M., de Kock, U., Saxby, H., and Repp, A.. (1985) 'An ecological comparison of small community-based houses and traditional institutions for severely and profoundly mentally handicapped adults: II Physical settings and the use of opportunities', *Behaviour Research and Therapy* 23: 337–48.

Felce, D., Saxby, H., de Kock, U., Repp, A., Ager, A., and Blunden, R. (1987) 'To what behaviours do attending adults respond?: a replication', *American Journal of Mental Deficiency* 91: 496–504.

Felce, D., Thomas, M., de Kock, U., Repp, A., Ager, A., and Blunden, R., (in press) 'Staff:client ratios and their effects on staff interactions and client behaviour in twelve facilities for severely and profoundly mentally handicapped adults', *Research in Developmental Disabilities.*

Goffman, E., (1961) *Asylums*, New York: Doubleday.

Griffiths, R., (1954) *The Abilities of Babies*, London: University of London Press.

——(1971) *The Abilities of Young Children*, Amersham: Association for Research in Infant and Child Development.

Humphreys, S., Lowe, K., and de Paiva, S. (1986) 'Long term evaluation of services for mentally handicapped people in Cardiff: progress report for 1985', Cardiff: Mental Handicap in Wales Applied Research Unit.

Jenkins, J., Felce, D., Toogood, S., Mansell, J., and de Kock, U. (in press) *Individual Programme Planning*, Kidderminster: BMIH Publications.

King, R., Raynes, N., and Tizard, J. (1971) *Patterns of Residential Care*, London: Routledge & Kegan Paul.

Kushlick, A. (1970) 'Residential care for the mentally subnormal', *Royal Society of Health Journal* 90: 255–61.

Landesman-Dwyer, S. (1981) 'Living in the community', *American Journal of Mental Deficiency* 86: 223–34.

——Sackett, G. P., and Kleinman, J. S. (1980) 'Relationship of size to resident and staff behaviour in small community residences', *American Journal of Mental Deficiency* 85: 6–17.

McBrien, J., and Weightman, J. (1980) 'The effect of room management procedures on the engagement of profoundly retarded children', *British Journal of Mental Subnormality*, 26: 38–46.
McKeown, T., Cross, K. W., and Keating, D. M. (1971) 'Influence of hospital siting on patient visiting', *Lancet*, 1082–6.
Mansell, J., Felce, D., de Kock, U., and Jenkins, J. (1982) 'Increasing purposeful activity of severely and profoundly mentally handicapped adults', *Behaviour Research and Therapy* 20: 593–604.
Mansell, J., Felce, D., Jenkins, J., de Kock, U., and Toogood, S., (1983) 'A Wessex home-from-home', *Nursing Times* 3 August: 51–6.
——(1987) *Developing Staffed Housing for People with Mental Handicaps*, Tunbridge Wells: Costello.
Mansell, J., Jenkins, J., Felce, D., and de Kock, U. (1984) 'Measuring the activity of severely and profoundly mentally handicapped adults in ordinary housing', *Behaviour Research and Therapy* 22: 23–9.
Mansell, J., Felce, D., Jenkins, J., Flight, C., and Dell, D. (1986) *The Bereweeke Skill-teaching System: Handbook*, 2nd edn, Windsor: National Foundation for Educational Research/Nelson Publishing Company.
Mathieson, S. and Blunden, R. (1980) 'Nimrod is piloting a course towards a community life', *Health and Social Service Journal* 90 25 Jan.: 122–4.
Moores, B. and Grant, G. W. B. (1976) 'On the nature and incidence of staff–patient interactions in hospitals for the mentally handicapped', *International Journal of Nursing Studies* 13: 69–81.
Morris, P. (1969) *Put Away*, London: Routledge & Kegan Paul.
Nihira, K., Foster, R., Shellhaus, M., and Leland, H. (1974) *AAMD Adaptive Behavior Scale*, Washington, DC: American Association of Mental Deficiency.
O'Brien, J. (1987) 'A guide to personal futures planning', in B. Wilcox and T. Bellamy (eds) *The Activities Catalog: An Alternative Curriculum for Youth and Adults with Severe Disabilities*, Baltimore: Paul H. Brookes Publishing Co.
O'Connor, N. and Tizard, J. (1951) 'Predicting the occupational adequacy of certified mental defectives', *Occupational Psychology* 25: 205–11.
——(1956) *The Social Problem of Mental Deficiency*, London: Pergamon.
Oswin, M. (1971) *The Empty Hours*, Harmondsworth: Penguin.
Porterfield, J., Blunden, R., and Blewitt, E. (1980) 'Improving environments for profoundly handicapped adults: using prompts and social attention to maintain high group engagement', *Behaviour Modification* 4: 225–41.
Repp, A. C. and Barton, L. E. (1980) 'Naturalistic observations of institutionalised retarded persons: a comparison of licensure decisions and behavioral observations', *Journal of Applied Behaviour Analysis* 13: 333–41.
——(1983) 'Naturalistic studies of retarded persons: functional relationships between the behaviour of staff and retarded persons', Department of Learning, Development and Special Education,

Northern Illinois University.
Reynell, J. K. (1977) *Reynell Developmental Language Scales*, Windsor: NFER–Nelson Publishing Co.
Saxby, H., Thomas, M., Felce, D., and de Kock, U., (1986) 'The use of shops, cafés and public houses by severely and profoundly mentally handicapped adults', *British Journal of Mental Subnormality* 32: 69–81.
Thomas, M., Felce, D., de Kock, U., Saxby, H., and Repp, A. C. (1986) 'The activity of staff and of severely and profoundly mentally handicapped adults in residential settings of different sizes', *British Journal of Mental Subnormality* 32: 82–92.
Thormahlen, P. W. (1965) 'A study of on-the-ward training of trainable mentally retarded children in a state institution', *California Mental Health Research Monograph*, no. 5.
Tizard, J. (1964) *Community Services for the Mentally Handicapped*, London: Oxford University Press.
Toogood, S., Jenkins, J., Felce, D., and de Kock, U. (1983) 'Opportunity plans', University of Southampton: Health Care Evaluation Research Team.
Ward, L. (1983) 'Mental handicap: an ordinary life', *Community Care*, 10 November.
Warren, S. A. and Mondy, L. W. (1971) 'To what behavior do attending adults respond?', *American Journal of Mental Deficiency* 75: 449–55.
Whatmore, R., Durward, L., and Kushlick, A. (1975) 'Measuring the quality of residential care', *Behavior Research and Therapy* 13: 227–36.
Wolfensberger, W. (1969) 'The origin and nature of our institutional models', in R. Kugel and W. Wolfensberger (eds) *Changing Patterns in Residential Services for the Mentally Retarded*, Washington, DC: President's Committee on Mental Retardation.
——(1972) *Normalisation: The Principle of Normalisation in Human Services*, Toronto: National Institute of Mental Retardation.
—— and Glenn, L. (1975) *Program Analysis of Service Systems: Handbook and Manual* 3rd edn, Toronto: National Institute on Mental Retardation.
Wright, E. C., Abbas, K. A., and Meredith, C. (1974) 'A study of the interactions between nursing staff and profoundly retarded children', *British Journal of Mental Subnormality* 20: 38.

Chapter Fifteen

THE EVALUATION OF THE ALL-WALES STRATEGY FOR PEOPLE WITH A MENTAL HANDICAP

GERRY EVANS, STUART TODD, AND STEPHEN BEYER

INTRODUCTION

In March 1983 the 'All-Wales Strategy for the Development of Services for Mentally Handicapped People' was published. In the introduction to the Strategy, the Secretary of State for Wales outlined that the aim was

> 'to correct the historic anomaly in the development of National Health Service and Local Authority provision which has left the bulk of public service provision in large, and for many, remote hospitals while the great majority of mentally handicapped people and their families receive little or no support in their home where it is most needed. The inadequacy of care in the community creates a cycle of dependence on institutional care because this is often the only option open to families who can no longer cope on their own.'
>
> (Welsh Office 1983)

The Strategy document provided guidance on new patterns of services for people with a mental handicap and for the preparation of detailed plans at the local level. The document was to be the 'touchstone for future developments in services' and was to be the basis on which the Welsh Office would consider the funding of future developments. The Strategy was to be implemented over a period of ten years with a commitment in 1983 of additional resources building up to £26 million per annum for community services.

The Strategy identified three philosophical principles which should guide its implementation, and emphasized that these principles should apply to all people with a mental handicap, however severe those handicaps.

(1) People with a mental handicap should have a right to normal patterns of life within the community.
(2) People with a mental handicap should have a right to be treated as individuals.
(3) People with a mental handicap require additional help from the communities in which they live and from professional services if they are to develop their maximum potential as individuals.

The Mental Handicap in Wales – Applied Research Unit of the University of Wales College of Medicine, and the Mental Handicap Project, University College of North Wales, were commissioned by the Welsh Office and the DHSS to undertake an evaluation of the All-Wales Strategy. This chapter provides a broad overview of the All-Wales Strategy, progress in its implementation, and an outline of the approach that the Mental Handicap in Wales Applied Research Unit is employing in the evaluation of the Strategy.

THE ALL-WALES STRATEGY

The All-Wales Strategy was launched following the recommendations of a working party report on services for people with a mental handicap (Welsh Office 1982). The working party's terms of reference were to prepare an outline for the development of an integrated pattern of comprehensive community-based services. The report was produced within a climate of concern regarding the lack of progress in the implementation of the ideas put forward on the White Paper *Better Services for the Mentally Handicapped* (DHSS 1971). There was particular concern with the rate of reduction of the number of people living in hospital. There was also an awareness that there existed a significant level of unmet need for services in the community.

The Strategy can be thought of as a value-led example of policy formulation in the sense that it defined objectives in terms of the nature of the lives of people with handicaps, rather than in terms of the types of services to be delivered. It was concerned not with setting down a blueprint by specifying concrete examples of future service development. Rather, it was concerned with the mobilization of 'human resources' in an effort to improve the quality of life of people with a mental handicap.

The principles, outlined above, formed the foundation of the Strategy. Although it has many components, the principles were seen as being central in the process of transforming service development and delivery. 'The principal measure of our success will be the extent to which we can say, after 10 years, that mentally handicapped people throughout Wales receive the respect and equal opportunities that are their due.' These principles are, first, that people with a mental handicap have a right to normal patterns of life. This principle not only reflects the view that people have a right to belong and participate in their communities, but more importantly, that 'they become respected members of their communities.' This statement illustrates the high standards that have been set by the Strategy, but is a recognition that the failure to set high standards will result in limited accomplishments. The second principle confirms the right of people with a mental handicap to be treated as individuals. This is a clear recognition that people are to be approached as having individual needs and aspirations. Services are no longer to offer blanket, impersonal responses but tailored opportunities that also involve a 'degree of adventure'. In addition, people with a mental handicap and their supporters were to become active partners in planning and making supported choices regarding their future. Finally, there is the recognition that in order to achieve their fullest potential, people will require additional help from their communities. This is not, as it may appear to be, a simple restatement of need, but represents a determination to create access to the resources and social networks of the community. Thus, there is a recognized need to encourage the participation of the community in achieving change.

The Strategy is then an attempt to develop a new pattern of services which reflect and safeguard the values on which it is based. Clearly, such principles do not translate easily into quantifiable service targets. They require services to be developed in a more responsive and innovative fashion. In order to achieve such change, two broad requirements of service co-ordination were specified. First, given the current structure of service delivery, with the dispersed allocation of responsibilities, the move towards flexibility requires a high degree of joint and effective planning between agencies. Second, the Strategy places considerable emphasis on building community services that are comprehensive in form and availability. It was stated that if new patterns of services were to achieve a high level of comprehensiveness, they should be able to demonstrate that they had:

- created access to a range of services that are available to the public – for example, housing; broadening the development of employment opportunities; creating maximum possible access to educational facilities; the availability of generic health care; provision for children in a range of services providing for children generally;
- developed a full range of support services – for example, the provision of support, advice, and teaching; the availability of a full range of short-term care programmes; a range of domiciliary services; planning and working with people with a mental handicap and their families;
- an integrated network of social and recreational opportunities – for example, building a planned network of volunteers; support of, and encouragement given to, the community in enabling people with mental handicap to blend with confidence into their communities;
- extensive planning and management arrangements, including co-operation between agencies; the development of the strength of the voluntary sector; the involvement of people with a mental handicap and their families in the planning of services;
- that no one through the level of their disability or their current situation should be excluded from the above – for example, that people with a mental handicap 'in hospital should not by virtue of that be given a second-class consideration'.

The existence of any services which aim to be as comprehensive as outlined above demands considerable co-operation between, and commitment from, different agencies. It also requires wide and extensive planning and management. The Strategy lays great emphasis on joint planning and management in bringing new services into being. This involves creating a partnership not only between statutory services, but also voluntary bodies and consumers. Great stress is also given to the development of advocacy schemes, the responsibility for such development being attributed to the voluntary sector.

Before the Welsh Office was prepared to release funds, all Welsh counties were to prepare and submit for approval plans on how they would pursue implementation. The Strategy laid down a challenge for service planners in that 'no one blue-print is prescribed for planning and management arrangements at the county level', but it was emphasized that Social Services Departments were to become the lead agency in the management of change. For the management of services at a more local level, the Strategy suggested a number of organizational concepts which might be relevant to local service delivery – for example, community mental handicap teams, key workers, and individual plans. In addition, at all levels of service planning, consumers were to be seen as essential partners.

When county plans had been approved by the Welsh Office, funds were then to be released. The working party had estimated the cost of providing comprehensive services as between £96 and £146 million per annum (1983–4 cash planning prices). It was estimated that there would be gross revenue saving arising from the transfer of people from hospitals to the community ranging from £2.8 to £17 million per annum, depending on the speed of reduction of hospital provision. The final suggested figure was therefore set at £112 million per annum.

At that time, agencies were spending approximately £32 million per annum on mental handicap services, the vast bulk of which was allocated to the health authorities. The Strategy stated that the full cost of £112 million could not reasonably be met by the Welsh Office. It was argued that the disparity between the estimated cost of the Strategy and annual expenditure on services in 1982 could be offset from revenue savings from the gradual run-down of traditional local authority services, – for example, hostels, and growth money and efficiency savings from health authorities. In addition, the Welsh Office would provide funding over the 10-year period of the Strategy, reaching a level of £26 million per annum in the tenth year. Although this would not provide the estimated £112 million, it was recognized that the change required would, given its radical nature, have to be gradual and incremental, and that it would be desirable 'to make the best use of experience before investing heavily'.

THE PROGRESS OF THE STRATEGY

Progress made in implementing the Strategy was to be monitored continuously, evaluated formally, and reviewed regularly. It was also emphasized that there should be an independent evaluation of the Strategy. The Welsh Office has recently completed its first review of the first 3 years of the Strategy (Welsh Office 1987). The Mental Handicap in Wales, Applied Research Unit has also, as part of its evaluation of the Strategy, conducted a review of issues resulting from the planning process in which counties have been engaged (Beyer et al. 1986). The main issues that have arisen from both these reviews are presented to provide a picture of progress to date in implementing the Strategy.

In the first two years of the Strategy the principal activity was planning, and the time it took to produce county plans varied across Wales. The Welsh Office had originally called on counties to submit plans for the implementation of the Strategy 6 months after its launch. This target was not met and five of the eight counties were asked to resubmit their plans. It was not until the end of 1985 that all counties had had their plans approved. The length of time taken reflected the influence of a number of factors. The Welsh Office adopted a firm role in ensuring that plans were of a high quality. A number of the counties experienced difficulties in setting up appropriate and effective structures to ensure the widest possible participation of a wide range of agencies and individuals in the planning process. Prior to the Strategy, there was some unease regarding previous experiences of joint planning. Although relations between authorities in many counties had been amicable, they had produced little in the way of effective, integrated planning. It was apparent that the process of plan formulation under the Strategy had effected improvements on previous efforts, and had produced genuine joint planning arrangements rather than merely plan consultation. By the end of the planning phase each county had established a planning mechanism, which included mechanisms for the management and co-ordination of service delivery. These were usually in the form of central or county groups, overseeing and unifying the work of local working groups (District or Area groups).

Since considerable time was given to the planning phase of the Strategy, progress in the development of new services was slower than originally anticipated. However, the Welsh Office in its review stated that a good start had been made in implementation. Early development had mainly focused on the development of domiciliary support and respite care schemes. The rate of provision of community-based accommodation for long-term living was slow. A number of factors appear to have obstructed major development in the field of accommodation provision, a key influence being the bureaucratic structures within local authorities.

Since the publication of the *Better Services* White Paper there have been attempts to shift the emphasis of responsibility for residential provision away from the health to the local authority sector. Although the Strategy is not a programme for hospital closure it is clear that considerable attention is paid to reviewing the role of health authority provision within mental handicap services. The Strategy states that admission to hospitals should be halted and that the resources and funds tied up in the health sector need to be transferred to community services. Progress on this front had also been slow with no major transfer of hospital residents to community settings and no evidence of the transfer of health authority monies to community services.

Between 1982 and 1985 the number of adults living in hospital fell by 8%, the number of children by 57%, an overall decrease of 9%. The number of admissions to hospitals in Wales increased over this period, although first admissions fell dramatically by 82%. These figures reflect the fact that the development of alternative living schemes has been insufficient to decrease significantly the size of the resident hospital population.

The proportion of mental handicap expenditure given to health authorities was, in 1983, 68% of total expenditure on mental handicap services. By 1985 the level had decreased to 60%. Meanwhile, the relative level of local authority expenditure had increased from 31% to 39% of total expenditure. Figure 15.1 shows the distribution of expenditure between different agencies and illustrates the allocation of additional Strategy funding in relation to total expenditure. The figure shows that Strategy funding was in 1985 10% of overall expenditure on mental handicap services. Between the period from 1983 to 1986 the amount of additional funds had risen from 2% to 10% of overall mental handicap expenditure, excluding education services.

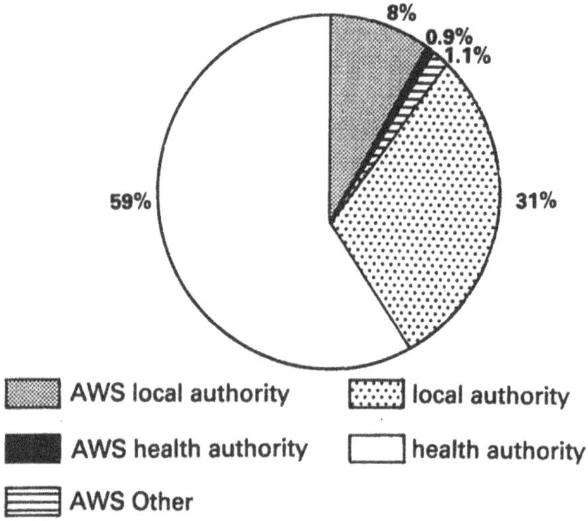

Figure 15.1 Expenditure on mental handicap services, 1985–6

The Strategy document did not provide detailed guidance on the intended role for education authorities, which led many to believe that the Strategy was a strategy for adults, not children. Moreover, the principles of the Strategy, if applied to children, suggested that education authorities would be providing services beyond their statutory obligations under the 1981 Act (Todd et al. 1987). A major problem identified in the reviews related to the role of education departments in the Strategy. In the majority of counties it was apparent that there was little evidence of the involvement of representatives of education in planning for the Strategy. Consequently, there was little in the plans submitted to the Welsh Office relating to developments in educational services to children. In particular, the issue of integrated education for children with handicaps had been largely ignored.

The All-Wales Strategy is a policy response to the problems faced by people with a mental handicap which sets high standards for those planning and delivering services. In addition, it has high expectations in terms of the change that needs to be achieved in the relationship between the people with handicaps and the communities in which they live. The Strategy has now been in operation for four years and although progress has been slower than expected, foundations have been established. As has been discussed there are a number of major obstacles to progress still in existence, largely arising from previous patterns of service delivery. Should these obstacles be overcome, major change should be possible.

EVALUATING THE AWS

The Mental Handicap in Wales Applied Research Unit was commissioned by the Welsh Office and the DHSS in 1984 to conduct an evaluation of the All-Wales Strategy. The programme of work for the evaluation involved a number of different phases of work. The main phases include a series of reviews of the processes involved in implementing the Strategy identifying the stages achieved at different points in time. Included in this phase of work is an analysis of the problems that have been encountered and particular successes that may have been achieved. Implementation is to be examined across Wales on a county basis and the first exercise was completed in 1985. This piece of work, highlighted above, examined progress made in producing plans for service development in each of the counties (Beyer et al. 1986). Another review is to be undertaken in 1989, analysing the development of new services on a county basis.

Another part of the evaluation is to involve a close examination of key components of the Strategy and this work is to begin in 1988. It will involve identification of good practice in sectors such as residential provision or day occupation and will involve the dissemination of lessons learnt in such sectors and working with service personnel in developing good practice in areas which appear to be in need of development.

The main part of the evaluation will, however, involve a detailed assessment of the impact of the All-Wales Strategy on the lives of people with a mental handicap in four districts within Wales. The rationale for this approach to the evaluation is that it may be possible to develop a whole range of plans, or even service structures, without having a major impact on the lives of the vast majority of people with handicaps. Clearly, it is possible to develop services which fail to have a positive impact on the major needs of service users. Although the Strategy explicitly states the positive impact that it is hoped to achieve for individuals, as Lakin et al. (1981) state

> The history of our society's policies regarding mentally retarded persons is replete with examples of how in the absence of systematic scrutiny, the sheer belief that what we are doing is appropriate, has led us to faithful adherence for years to counterproductive treatment models.

Increasingly, policy documents are making explicit the values which underpin service delivery by specifying the desired outcomes for service users. As has been shown, the All-Wales Strategy is firmly based on a set of principles regarding the desired position of people with handicaps in society and has translated these into a set of objectives. In having specific objectives against which to evaluate the success, or otherwise, of the Strategy, the task of the evaluator should be easier. However, the development of evaluation in Britain has been firmly linked to policy development with new techniques of evaluation usually having been developed in response to developments in patterns of service delivery (Evans et al. 1988). Changes in patterns of service delivery have however been particularly rapid and radical in recent years. This has left evaluators with a major challenge in developing new methods that will adequately assess the impact, and success, of the new services. Evaluative research has historically been ineffective in devising measures that accurately measure outcomes of service inputs in ways that are also meaningful to the lives of service users.

Policy documents such as the All-Wales Strategy have gone further in defining objectives in terms of the position of people with handicaps in relation to the communities in which they live, i.e. outcomes which cannot be exclusively linked to service inputs. If evaluation is to assess the effectiveness of services, or policy strategies, in meaningful terms, there must be a social context to the evaluation which relates service inputs to a broader analysis of the lives of service users. The challenge for those evaluating human services must be, therefore, to develop measures which accurately describe the life experiences of individuals and which can also monitor changes in the quality of people's experiences over time.

There is a need, therefore, to introduce evaluative criteria which are not based in the culture of service delivery, but rather criteria which are related to wider societal standards. The ideology of normalization which has been developed over the last 20 years provides an analysis of the difficulties faced by people who are handicapped or elderly in social terms. While no reference is made in the Strategy document to the ideology of normalization, it can be considered as a policy document that contains most of the fundamental principles of normalization. Included in the objectives of the Strategy is the statement that people with a mental handicap 'should be enabled to become respected members of their communities and should not be devalued because of their intellectual impairment'. This objective embodies the main goal of the normalization philosophy.

In its evaluation of the All-Wales Strategy the Mental Handicap in Wales Applied Research Unit has adopted an approach which combines a number of techniques that have been employed in normalization-related work. In particular, the framework for conceptualizing the evaluation has drawn on normalization-related concepts. Emerson and Pretty (1987) identify important principles which could act as a basis for the development of measures. They include as one of their main principles the need to relate the situation of the person with a handicap to the wider culture in which they live. Work done at the University of Uppsala by the Mental Retardation Project (Kebbon 1982) has attempted to operationalize some of the concepts of normalization by developing an analysis of the process of the integration of people with handicaps into natural communities. The stages analysed are those of, first, the extent to which people are physically located in ordinary communities, second, the extent to which individuals actively participate within their communities, and finally, the extent of satisfaction that people express regarding their lives.

The Unit has decided to concentrate its efforts on evaluating the extent to which people are physically and socially integrated. At present, it has been decided that a further stage of analysis will not be undertaken. This further stage would involve an assessment of the satisfaction of service users with their life-styles, and also some means of assessing whether the community perception of people with handicaps has been enhanced as a result of greater contact. Evidence from research studies in the United States

(Butler and Bjannes 1978) have shown that the process of social integration is a very slow one and therefore, the period of research funding will probably only allow for an examination of the effect of the Strategy in achieving a degree of integration.

The approach employed for the evaluation has also drawn on the work done on service accomplishments (O'Brien in press) and service goals (Kristiansen and Ness 1988). As O'Brien states, 'The history of philosophy offers many attempts at understanding what people mean by quality of life. Each is indicative; none is definitive.' He goes on to identify what he defines as five essential accomplishments as a means of examining the quality of a person's life experiences. The five areas identified by O'Brien are community presence, choice, competence, respect, and community participation. Kristiansen (1988) has developed the ideas of O'Brien and included in the goals that should be achieved for individuals those of expression and recognition of individuality and the experience of continuity in one's life. These areas were used as a basis in identifying an approach to examining the current life experiences of individuals and the evaluation of whether change occurs over a 3-year period.

The Unit has employed a survey-based approach to the evaluation collecting information on 58 per cent of the people with a mental handicap living in, or originally from, four geographically and culturally varied districts in south and west Wales. Interviews have been conducted with relatives and staff and, where possible, people with a mental handicap, using a structured questionnaire specifically designed and piloted for the evaluation (Evans et al. 1988). The questionnaire was designed to obtain information on the following areas:

(1) *Social background:* information on the demographic characteristics of individuals, their place of residence, including information on whom people live with. For those individuals living at home, details of the social and economic characteristics of the households are obtained.
(2) *Degree of dependency:* a broad picture is obtained of the abilities of individuals, including information on their medical health.
(3) *Personal growth:* information on the persons ability to undertake key community activities and also an attempt to discover whether individuals are in environments where they

are expected to develop and given opportunities to do so.

(4) *Links with support networks:* the extent of contact that individuals have with specialist and generic services, and information on the existence and nature of informal supports.

(5) *Day occupation:* the amount of time the person spends in organized day services or in full-time, part-time, or voluntary employment.

(6) *Future planning:* the nature of mechanisms employed for planning futures with the person with the handicap. Included is information on the process employed and on the type of options available to the individual.

(7) *Networks and relationships:* the number and nature of close friendships and acquaintanceships with community citizens.

(8) *Community activities* the range of activities undertaken, with information on frequency, settings for activities, and who else shares in the activities.

(9) *Status:* information on the domains of an individual's life which allow for expression of choice and identity.

The evaluation is to take place over a 3-year period with the first round of data collection having been conducted in four districts in late 1986 and early 1987, with information having been obtained on 512 individuals. Areas were selected to reflect cultural and geographical variations. The four areas chosen were Ceredigion district in West Wales, the Rhondda valleys, East Gwent, and one Social Services area in inner Swansea.

Ceredigion is a predominantly rural area which has retained a strong Welsh-speaking culture. Its coastal location has, however, resulted in high levels of in-migration from England. The Rhondda valleys are in the classic South Wales coal-mining tradition. The valleys are comprised of largely terraced housing and, with the decline of the coal industry, high levels of unemployment and deprivation are present. East Gwent is again a predominantly rural area, but being located on the English borders, its culture can be viewed as anglicized. It is also one of the most affluent parts of Wales in terms of a range of indicators, including income levels and housing patterns. The area of Swansea included in the survey is characteristic of most urban areas, with a highly mobile population in the most central areas, and a more stable population in suburban areas.

The population for the study were those people with a mental handicap aged 5 or over who lived in, or came from, the district in which the study was to be conducted. Only those people coming from the district but living in residential services outside of Wales were excluded. The basis for this exclusion was that the person would not be receiving or benefiting from services directed under the All-Wales Strategy. All individuals identified as being originally from the four districts but who were living in residential services within Wales were included.

The design of the evaluation, as outlined above, involves a second data collection point, 3 years after the first. In order to measure the impact of the Strategy over this period, it was necessary to derive statistically appropriate sample sizes. This was achieved largely through the analysis of data collected during developmental work on the evaluation. It was calculated that a sample size of 50% would be adequate. However, an additional 10% was added to this figure to insure against people not wishing or being able to participate at second data collection point.

In total 512 interviews were conducted, or 58% of the combined register populations for the four districts. These interviews were conducted from a targeted base of 632, representing, therefore, an 81% response rate. The percentage sample size is slightly below the intended size of 60%, but the final sample size of 58% is within the margins of safety for measuring the extent of change over three years.

A strong emphasis is placed in the evaluation on feeding back the results of the survey work to service personnel and service users in each of the districts concerned. The approach employed for the feedback involves, first, describing the district in terms of variables such as geography, culture, and employment patterns, this information being obtained from census returns and from local planning authority documents. This is followed by a description of the population of people with a mental handicap in the district in terms of age, sex, and current residence, obtained from local registers or lists held by local service personnel. The results of the survey are then presented in terms of a description of the current situation of people with handicaps in, or originally from, the district. An analysis is then presented of the extent to which the objectives of the Strategy are being met in terms of the participation of people with handicaps in their communities. Both a verbal and written feedback is given, with a report being produced on each of the districts and an overall report produced analysing trends across the four districts which examines more broadly the situation of people with a mental handicap in today's society.

The All-Wales Strategy provides a unique opportunity for evaluators to implement new forms of evaluation attempting to relate the experiences of people with a mental handicap to the communities in which they live. This chapter has set out an outline of the basis for such an approach to evaluation, and has described briefly the approach employed in evaluating the Strategy. The Strategy is an attempt to develop new forms of community-based services which are designed radically to improve the quality of life of people with a mental handicap. It states clearly the kind of change that is required in terms of the experiences of people with a handicap rather than prescribing the nature of the services to be delivered. As has been discussed, however, the Strategy has met serious obstacles early in its implementation which have delayed progress in major areas of service development, for example in the availability of housing. However, should these obstacles be overcome, the preliminary work done in planning for and implementing the Strategy could form a basis for major change. The initial analysis of data collected from the first phase of the evaluation reveals that there is still considerable progress to be made in meeting the objectives of the Strategy in achieving valued social roles for people with a mental handicap in their communities.

REFERENCES

Beyer, S., Evans, G., Todd, S., and Blunden, R. (1986) *Planning for the All-Wales Strategy: A Review of Issues Arising in Welsh Counties*, Cardiff: Mental Handicap in Wales – Applied Research Unit.

Butler, E. W. and Bjannes, A. T. (1978) 'Activities and use of time by retarded persons in community care facilities', in G. P. Sacket (ed.) *Observing Behaviour (vol. 1): Theory and Applications in Mental Retardation*, Baltimore: University Park Press.

DHSS (1970) *Better Services for the Mentally Handicapped*, Cmnd. 4683, London: HMSO.

Emerson, E. B. and Pretty, G. M. H. (1987) 'Enhancing the social relevance of evaluation practice'. *Disability, Handicap and Society* 2: 151–62.

Evans, G., Beyer, S., and Todd, S. (1988) 'Looking forward not looking back: the evaluation of community living'. *Disability, Handicap and Society* 3(3): 239–52.

Kebbon, L. (1982) *Normalisation in Sweden: Quality and Limitations*, Psychiatric Research Center, University of Uppsala, Sweden: Mental Retardation Project.

Kristiansen, K. and Ness, N. E. (1988) *Hjelpesystemet: I gar, I dag, I morgon*, Trondeim: University of Trondeim.

Lakin, K. C., Bruininks, R. H., and Sigford, B. B. (1981) 'Deinstitutionalisation and community adjustment: a summary of research and issues', in R. H. Bruininks, C. E. Meyers, B. B. Sigford, and K. C. Lakin (eds) *Deinstitutionalisation and Community Adjustment of Mentally Retarded People*, American Association on Mental Deficiency.

O'Brien, J. (in press) 'A guide to personal futures planning', in G. T. Bellamy and B. Wilcox (eds) *The Activities Catalog: A Community Programming Guide for Youth and Adults with Severe Disabilities*, Baltimore: Brookes.

Todd, S., Beyer, S., and Evans, G. (1987) 'The All Wales Strategy and the education of children with severe mental handicap', *Mental Handicap* 15: 22–5.

Welsh Office (1982) *Report of the All Wales Working Party on Services for Mentally Handicapped People*, Cardiff: Welsh Office.

——(1983) *The All Wales Strategy for the Development of Services for Mentally Handicapped People*, Cardiff: Welsh Office.

——(1987) *The All Wales Strategy for the Development of Services for Mentally Handicapped People. A Review of Progress since March 1983*, Cardiff: Welsh Office.

Chapter Sixteen

CONCLUSIONS AND IMPLICATIONS

SARA BARNA

Concluding a series of contributions as varied as those in the foregoing chapters is inevitably subjective, but there appear to be some recurring themes and issues which colour the debate.

In recent years, the political context has clearly been generally supportive of community care and the move away from large-scale institutional forms of care. However, as the real costs of good-quality community care become apparent, there is already evidence of a decreasing political impetus. There is no doubt that community care is being provided on the cheap in some places and many people are pessimistic about the prospects for future funding. On the other hand, many of the papers collected here reflect considerable optimism about future services and what it is possible to achieve. The gap between optimists and pessimists is not solely connected with funding. Whilst it is not possible to achieve high-quality services without adequate resources, there are also other issues of major importance concerning organizational structures in particular. Individual projects vary enormously on such dimensions as, for example, the amount of organizational support they receive (both in terms of management support for policy and practice issues and social support) and also in their perceived status, both locally and nationally. High-quality services cannot be developed, let alone maintained, when many of the personnel attempting to provide them are working in relative isolation within generally unsupportive organizational structures.

In terms of planning services, it is clear that fundamentally different models exist in relation to resettlement from long-stay hospitals. One of the themes that emerged is how much can or should people be prepared or 'rehabilitated' before they move away from the institutions. Some projects involve a large number of small steps in preparing people for gradual transition from institutional to ordinary living. Others do not involve such intermediate stages but essentially comprise a move direct from an institution to an ordinary house for the individual. The differences in strategy appear to be partly, but by no means entirely, related to different client groups, with the former being more typical of services for people recovering from mental illness and the latter more commonly found in services for people with mental handicaps. The different models and resultant strategies would appear to reflect differences in the underlying assumptions and philosophies which may or may not be made explicit. The 'small steps' model would appear to reflect two underlying assumptions. First, that there is a stress factor involved in moving out of a long-stay hospital and the finely graded approach is designed to minimize this and thereby avoid breakdown and failure; and second, that the individual has to meet certain criteria in order to live in the community and services are therefore geared to supporting people in attaining such standards. A further assumption is that some people will not reach the criteria and there will therefore be a continuing need for asylum. At the other extreme, the assumption is that everyone has the right to live in the community and the aim of services should therefore be to support them in so doing, regardless of the degree of disability or the challenge they present to service providers. Following on from such assumptions, some projects would tend to concentrate first on helping the least disabled or challenging people to move, whilst others would view such an approach as both unnecessary and undesirable. In this context, it is worth noting that several contributors to the conference commented on the general drift of service provision from more seriously to less seriously disabled people.

Community care is, of course, not just about resettlement from long-stay hospitals but about people already living in the community. Although the focus of much attention is on people leaving long-stay hospitals to return to the community, it must be remembered that the vast majority of people with special needs have always been cared for within their local communities, largely through informal and unpaid care networks (Equal Opportunities Commission 1982). One concern is that the reallocation of resources to the 'new community services' will result in little or no improvement in the generally inadequate level of services for people already in the community. At the same time, it appears that it will be difficult to maintain what are already widely acknowledged to be inadequate services within the contracting institutions. Whilst there are many examples of good practice within community services, and one of the aims of this collection of papers has been to highlight some of these, it is also apparent that very different standards of quality are emerging. It seems likely that the discrepancies will increase between some well-planned and funded 'new' community projects, poorly funded and largely informal existing community care arrangements, and increasingly under-funded and demoralized institutional care.

One important issue concerns the future of institutions. In recent years there have often been debates as to definitions of 'the community' and what living 'in the community' means. Conversely, there are sometimes difficulties in thinking clearly about institutions. Obviously, the size of institutions alone militates against any attempt to provide high-quality care, but size is not the only problem. A number of contributors warned of the dangers of creating new smaller institutions physically located within 'the community' but which do little to enhance the quality of people's lives. Another point to consider is that institutions were created to meet certain needs. The changing philosophies and fashions in relation to human services have been well documented elsewhere (for example, Foucault 1965), but one aim of institutional care had been to provide asylum in the sense of sanctuary or refuge. In our enthusiasm for integration and progress, it may be important to remember this and to aim to maintain this option for some people, whilst also striving to improve models of care within such institutions. One of the concerns is that new developments in the community are often dependent in terms of funding on institutions contracting. This situation appears to further widen the scope for friction and conflict and to contribute to decreasing morale within institutions. It also means that there can be the danger of people losing out on services, stranded between traditional services in the process of being dismantled and new services which are not yet established. The need for bridging funding to alleviate this has been widely recognized in the field but has not been acted upon. Finally, several contributors acknowledge that, given the current pace of community care developments, institutions are likely to remain with us in the foreseeable future. It is therefore essential to find ways of maintaining and raising standards within such traditional services, at the same time as developing new community-based services.

In the current climate of transitional services there are competing and conflicting ideologies and models of care, as well as some people with more obvious vested interests, who stand to lose or gain according to the shifts in resources. There is an assumption that basic values are shared, but whilst this may generally be true, it is also important to recognize that there will be other agendas concerning, for example, the erosion of power, protection of jobs, and fear of change. In this context it is not surprising that debates are often highly emotionally charged and, in consequence, working relationships between different agencies, between disciplines, and between individuals, can at times become extremely fraught and stressful.

It is important to note that most of the public debate on community care has taken place within the circles of professionals employed by the statutory services and politicians, the voluntary sector also having some voice. Consumers or service users are rarely heard, although lip-service is frequently paid to their involvement. In addition, there is often confusion between the primary consumers and carers, or secondary consumers, whose needs are not necessarily the same.

One of the major issues in relation to the contraction of long-stay hospitals concerns the staff who are currently employed. Morale within such institutions is understandably extremely low, with little prospect of any significant improvement. One of the points which is currently debated is whether or not staff who trained and work within traditional services will be able to transfer to the emerging community services. There are particular issues concerning shifts in philosophy, attitudes, and skills. There are for example, situations in which hospital staff have transferred to new community services but, because they have not been involved in the planning process, they have little idea of the values and philosophies which shape the new developments. There are also situations in which new community services have been planned and implemented by personnel with no direct experience with a particular client group, and the knowledge and experience of staff within the institution has been lost. There are also many practical issues, such as geographical factors and conditions of service, which need to be addressed in relation to the transfer of staff. As stated clearly in an earlier chapter, staff training issues cannot be seen in isolation but must be viewed as an integral part of overall service planning and development.

A main aim of the conference on which this book is based was to bring together people working with different client groups. Many issues, including those arising from the contraction of hospitals, arise in similar ways for different client groups, yet there is relatively little interchange across the conventional service groupings of mental handicap, mental illness, and services to elderly people. It would seem that there should be scope for much fruitful collaboration and interchange at a number of levels, from broad planning issues through to very specific practical details. However, it is evident that different professional cultures are associated with the different client- based service groupings and some people feel the differences are too great. Whilst such differences may make genuine interchange difficult to achieve, it is also a greater reason to attempt to increase the contact between service providers in order that lessons may be learnt to the benefit of future service users. In general, it is difficult to find an appropriate forum in which such interchange might occur. It would appear that the current political climate encourages management structures and styles which tend to be competitive and insular and thus perhaps unwittingly contribute to a lack of exchange at practitioner level. In the absence of structural solutions it would therefore seem that professionals in the field need to seek informal means and structures to facilitate interchange.

REFERENCES

Equal Opportunities Commission (1982) *Research Report*, Equal Opportunities Commission, Overseas House, Key Street, Manchester M3 3HN.

Foucault, M. (1965) *Madness and Civilisation – a History of Insanity in the Age of Reason*, London: Tavistock Publications

NAME INDEX

SUBJECT INDEX

For Product Safety Concerns and Information please contact our
EU representative GPSR@taylorandfrancis.com Taylor & Francis
Verlag GmbH, Kaufingerstraße 24, 80331 München, Germany